Introduction

In a world where masculinity is often associated with hearty portions and bold flavors, the journey towards optimal health can sometimes feel like uncharted territory for men. But fear not, for **_"Manly Meals for Gut Health"_** is here to redefine what it means to eat like a man while prioritizing gut health.

This cookbook is not just about following the latest food trends or adhering to restrictive diets. Instead, it's a celebration of flavorful, satisfying meals crafted specifically with men's nutritional needs in mind. With over 100 meticulously curated recipes, each dish is thoughtfully designed to nourish the body from within, supporting digestive health and overall well-being.

From savory breakfast options that kickstart the day with energy to hearty dinners that satisfy even the most robust appetites, every recipe in this book is a testament to the idea that eating well doesn't mean sacrificing flavor or masculinity. Whether you're a seasoned chef or a novice in the kitchen, you'll find something to tantalize your taste buds and invigorate your gut.

But **_"Manly Meals for Gut Health"_** is more than just a collection of recipes. It's a guide to understanding the intricate connection between what we eat and how we feel, empowering men to take control of their health and make informed choices about the foods they consume. With insights into the importance of gut health and practical tips for incorporating gut-friendly ingredients into everyday meals, this book is a valuable resource for anyone looking to prioritize their well-being.

So, grab your apron and get ready to embark on a culinary adventure that combines the best of bold flavors and gut-nourishing ingredients. "Manly Meals for Gut Health" is not just a cookbook – it's a roadmap to a healthier, happier you.

1. Greek yogurt with honey and berries

Ingredients:
- 1 cup plain Greek yogurt
- 1-2 tablespoons honey
- 1/2 cup fresh berries (such as blueberries, raspberries, or strawberries)

Instructions:

1. Scoop the Greek yogurt into a bowl.

2. Drizzle the honey over the top of the yogurt.

3. Gently fold the honey into the yogurt until it is well combined.

4. Top the yogurt with the fresh berries.

That's it! The cool, creamy Greek yogurt paired with the sweet honey and juicy berries makes for a delicious and healthy breakfast or snack. You can adjust the amounts of honey and berries to your taste preferences. Enjoy!

2. Overnight oats with chia seeds and almond milk

Ingredients:
- 1/2 cup rolled oats
- 1 tablespoon chia seeds
- 1/2 cup unsweetened almond milk
- 1 tablespoon maple syrup or honey (optional)
- 1/4 teaspoon vanilla extract (optional)
- Pinch of cinnamon (optional)
- Fresh fruit for topping (such as berries, sliced banana, etc.)

Instructions:
1. In a mason jar or other airtight container, combine the rolled oats and chia seeds.

2. Pour in the almond milk and stir to combine.

3. If using, stir in the maple syrup/honey, vanilla, and cinnamon.

4. Seal the container and refrigerate overnight, or for at least 4-6 hours.

5. In the morning, give the oats a stir. They should have thickened up nicely.

6. Top with your desired fresh fruit.

That's it! The chia seeds and oats will soak up the almond milk overnight, creating a creamy, pudding-like texture. The chia seeds also provide extra fiber and nutrients. You can customize the toppings to your liking. Enjoy this easy, make-ahead breakfast!

3. Smoothie bowl with spinach, banana, and flax seeds

Ingredients:
- 1 cup unsweetened almond milk (or milk of your choice)
- 1 frozen banana
- 1 cup fresh spinach
- 1 tablespoon ground flax seeds
- 1 tablespoon honey or maple syrup (optional)
- Toppings (such as sliced banana, berries, granola, nut butter, etc.)

Instructions:

1. In a high-powered blender, combine the almond milk, frozen banana, spinach, and flax seeds.

2. Blend on high speed until the mixture is smooth and creamy, about 1-2 minutes.

3. If desired, add the honey or maple syrup and blend again briefly to incorporate.

4. Pour the smoothie into a bowl.

5. Top with your desired toppings, such as sliced banana, berries, granola, nut butter, etc.

The frozen banana helps create a thick, creamy texture, while the spinach adds a boost of nutrients. The flax seeds provide fiber and healthy omega-3 fatty acids. Feel free to adjust the amounts of each ingredient to suit your taste preferences.

This smoothie bowl makes for a nutritious and satisfying breakfast or snack. Enjoy!

4. Avocado toast with a poached egg

Ingredients:
- 2 slices of whole grain or sourdough bread
- 1 ripe avocado, mashed
- 1 tablespoon olive oil
- 1 tablespoon lemon juice
- Salt and pepper to taste
- 2 eggs
- Vinegar (for poaching the eggs)

Instructions:

1. Toast the bread slices until lightly golden.

2. In a small bowl, mash the avocado with the olive oil, lemon juice, salt, and pepper until well combined.

3. Spread the mashed avocado evenly over the toasted bread slices.

4. Bring a medium saucepan of water to a gentle simmer and add a splash of vinegar. Crack the eggs one at a time into the simmering water and poach for 3-4 minutes, until the whites are set but the yolks are still runny.

5. Using a slotted spoon, carefully transfer the poached eggs on top of the avocado toast.

6. Season the poached eggs with a pinch of salt and pepper.

Enjoy your avocado toast with the perfectly poached egg on top. The creamy avocado, tangy lemon, and runny egg yolk make for a delicious and satisfying breakfast or snack.

You can customize this recipe by adding additional toppings like diced tomatoes, crumbled feta, or a sprinkle of red pepper flakes.

5. Oatmeal with apples and cinnamon

Ingredients:
- 1 cup old-fashioned rolled oats
- 2 cups unsweetened almond milk (or milk of your choice)
- 1 medium apple, peeled, cored, and diced
- 1 teaspoon ground cinnamon
- 1 tablespoon honey or maple syrup (optional)
- Pinch of salt

Instructions:

1. In a medium saucepan, combine the rolled oats and almond milk. Bring the mixture to a simmer over medium heat, stirring occasionally.

2. Once the oats have started to thicken, about 5 minutes, stir in the diced apple, cinnamon, and a pinch of salt.

3. Continue cooking the oatmeal, stirring frequently, until it reaches your desired consistency, about 5-7 minutes more.

4. If using, stir in the honey or maple syrup.

5. Serve the oatmeal warm, garnished with additional cinnamon, apple slices, or any other desired toppings.

The apples and cinnamon add a delicious, autumnal flavor to the creamy oatmeal. The honey or maple syrup can be added for extra sweetness, if desired.

This oatmeal makes for a comforting and nutritious breakfast. You can adjust the amount of liquid and cooking time to achieve your preferred texture. Enjoy!

6. Whole grain pancakes with kefir

Ingredients:
- 1 cup whole wheat flour
- 1/2 cup all-purpose flour
- 2 teaspoons baking powder
- 1/2 teaspoon baking soda
- 1/4 teaspoon salt
- 1 cup kefir
- 1/2 cup milk
- 1 egg
- 2 tablespoons honey or maple syrup
- 1 teaspoon vanilla extract
- Butter or oil for cooking

Instructions:

1. In a large bowl, whisk together the whole wheat flour, all-purpose flour, baking powder, baking soda, and salt.

2. In a separate bowl, whisk together the kefir, milk, egg, honey/maple syrup, and vanilla.

3. Pour the kefir mixture into the dry ingredients and stir just until combined (do not overmix).

4. Heat a large skillet or griddle over medium heat and lightly grease with butter or oil.

5. Scoop about 1/4 cup of the batter onto the hot surface, cooking in batches as needed.
6. Cook the pancakes for 2-3 minutes per side, or until golden brown.

7. Serve the pancakes warm, with additional kefir, honey, fruit, or other desired toppings.

The kefir in these pancakes adds a nice tangy flavor and helps create a light, fluffy texture. The whole wheat flour boosts the fiber and nutrient content. Feel free to adjust the sweetener to your taste preferences.

These wholesome pancakes make for a delicious and satisfying breakfast. Enjoy!

7. Scrambled eggs with spinach and tomatoes

Ingredients:
- 6 large eggs
- 2 tablespoons milk or water
- 1 tablespoon butter or olive oil
- 1 cup fresh spinach, chopped
- 1 cup cherry tomatoes, halved
- 2 tablespoons grated Parmesan cheese (optional)
- Salt and pepper to taste

Instructions:

1. In a medium bowl, whisk together the eggs and milk/water until well combined.

2. Heat a nonstick skillet over medium heat and melt the butter or heat the olive oil.

3. Add the chopped spinach to the skillet and cook for 1-2 minutes, until slightly wilted.

4. Pour the egg mixture into the skillet and let it sit for 20-30 seconds to set the bottom.

5. Using a spatula, gently push the eggs from the side of the pan towards the center, tilting the pan to allow the uncooked egg to flow to the edges.

6. Once the eggs are mostly set but still look a bit wet, stir in the halved cherry tomatoes.

7. Continue cooking and stirring the eggs until they reach your desired doneness, about 2-3 minutes total.

8. Remove the skillet from heat and stir in the Parmesan cheese, if using.

9. Season the scrambled eggs with salt and pepper to taste.

10. Serve the scrambled eggs with spinach and tomatoes immediately.

The spinach and tomatoes add color, flavor, and extra nutrition to these fluffy scrambled eggs. The Parmesan cheese is optional but adds a nice savory touch. Enjoy this healthy and delicious breakfast!

8. Chia pudding with mango

Ingredients:
- 1/2 cup chia seeds
- 2 cups unsweetened almond milk (or milk of your choice)
- 2 tablespoons honey or maple syrup
- 1 teaspoon vanilla extract
- 1 ripe mango, peeled and diced

Instructions:

1. In a medium bowl, whisk together the chia seeds, almond milk, honey/maple syrup, and vanilla extract until well combined.

2. Cover the bowl and refrigerate for at least 4 hours, or overnight, stirring occasionally, until the chia seeds have thickened the mixture into a pudding-like consistency.

3. Once the chia pudding has set, divide it into serving bowls or jars.

4. Top each serving with the diced mango.

5. Optionally, you can add additional toppings like toasted coconut, chopped nuts, or a drizzle of extra honey.

The chia seeds will absorb the liquid and create a thick, creamy pudding. The sweet, tropical mango pairs beautifully with the nutty chia flavor.

This chia pudding makes for a nutritious and satisfying breakfast or snack. The prep time is minimal, and you can make it ahead of time for easy grab-and-go meals throughout the week. Enjoy!

9. Buckwheat porridge with walnuts and blueberries

Ingredients:
- 1 cup raw buckwheat groats
- 3 cups unsweetened almond milk (or milk of your choice)
- 1 tablespoon maple syrup (or honey)
- 1/4 teaspoon ground cinnamon
- 1/4 cup chopped walnuts
- 1 cup fresh or frozen blueberries

Instructions:

1. In a medium saucepan, combine the buckwheat groats and almond milk. Bring the mixture to a boil over medium-high heat.

2. Once boiling, reduce the heat to low, cover the saucepan, and let the buckwheat simmer for 10-15 minutes, stirring occasionally, until the groats are tender and the porridge has thickened.

3. Remove the saucepan from heat and stir in the maple syrup and cinnamon until well combined.

4. Divide the buckwheat porridge into serving bowls.

5. Top each serving with chopped walnuts and fresh or frozen blueberries.

The nutty, earthy flavor of the buckwheat pairs beautifully with the sweet blueberries and crunchy walnuts. The maple syrup and cinnamon add warmth and depth to the porridge.

Buckwheat is a gluten-free grain that is high in fiber, protein, and various vitamins and minerals. This porridge makes for a nutritious and satisfying breakfast or brunch.

Feel free to adjust the sweetener, spices, and toppings to your personal taste preferences. Enjoy this wholesome and delicious buckwheat porridge!

10. Whole grain cereal with unsweetened almond milk

Ingredients:
- 1 cup whole grain cereal (such as oats, quinoa, or a mixed whole grain blend)
- 1 cup unsweetened almond milk

Instructions:

1. Pour the whole grain cereal into a bowl.
2. Pour the unsweetened almond milk over the cereal.
3. Stir gently to combine.

That's it! This is a basic but nutritious breakfast option.

Some tips and variations:

- Choose a whole grain cereal that is low in added sugars. Look for options that have minimal or no added sweeteners.

- You can use any type of unsweetened plant-based milk, such as oat milk or cashew milk, in place of the almond milk.

- Top the cereal with fresh fruit, such as berries, sliced banana, or diced apple, for added flavor and nutrition.

- Sprinkle on some nuts, seeds, or a drizzle of honey or maple syrup for extra texture and sweetness.

- For a creamier texture, you can let the cereal sit in the milk for a few minutes before eating.

This simple whole grain cereal with almond milk makes for a quick, healthy, and satisfying breakfast. Adjust the portions to suit your appetite.

11. Quinoa breakfast bowl with nuts and dried fruits

Ingredients:
- 1 cup quinoa, rinsed
- 2 cups milk of your choice (dairy, almond, etc.)
- 1 tsp vanilla extract
- 1/4 tsp ground cinnamon
- Pinch of salt
- 1/4 cup slivered almonds
- 1/4 cup walnut halves
- 1/4 cup dried cranberries or cherries
- 2 tbsp honey or maple syrup
- Fresh fruit like bananas, berries, etc. (optional)

Instructions:

1. In a saucepan, combine the quinoa and milk. Bring to a boil over medium-high heat.

2. Reduce heat to low, add the vanilla, cinnamon and salt. Simmer for 15-20 minutes, stirring occasionally, until quinoa is fluffy and liquid is absorbed.

3. Remove quinoa from heat and let stand for 5 minutes, covered. Fluff with a fork.

4. Transfer cooked quinoa to a bowl. Top with the slivered almonds, walnut halves, dried cranberries/cherries and a drizzle of honey or maple syrup.

5. Optional: Add fresh sliced bananas, berries or other fruits on top.

6. You can warm up the nuts and dried fruits by heating them briefly in a pan if desired.

7. Serve the quinoa breakfast bowls warm. Add extra milk if you prefer a thinner, porridge-like consistency.

This nutty, fruity quinoa bowl makes a hearty, protein-packed breakfast. Feel free to mix up the nut varieties and dried fruits you use. You can also substitute the milk for water or broth if preferred. Quinoa is nutritious and filling!

12. Grilled chicken salad with mixed greens and vinaigrette

Ingredients:
Salad:
- 4 boneless, skinless chicken breasts
- 5 oz mixed greens
(such as spinach, arugula, and kale)
- 1 cup cherry tomatoes, halved
- 1/2 cucumber, sliced
- 1/4 red onion, thinly sliced

Vinaigrette:
- 2 tablespoons olive oil
- 1 tablespoon balsamic vinegar
- 1 teaspoon Dijon mustard
- 1 teaspoon honey
- Salt and pepper to taste

Instructions:
1. Preheat your grill or grill pan to medium-high heat.

2. Season the chicken breasts with salt and pepper.

3. Grill the chicken for 5-7 minutes per side, or until cooked through. Allow to rest for 5 minutes, then slice or chop the chicken.

4. In a large salad bowl, combine the mixed greens, cherry tomatoes, cucumber, and red onion.

5. In a small bowl, whisk together the olive oil, balsamic vinegar, Dijon mustard, and honey. Season the vinaigrette with salt and pepper to taste.

6. Drizzle the vinaigrette over the salad and toss to coat.

7. Top the salad with the grilled chicken slices.

Serve the grilled chicken salad immediately. The combination of the tender, flavorful chicken, fresh greens, and tangy vinaigrette makes for a delicious and nutritious meal.

You can customize this salad by adding other toppings, such as avocado, crumbled feta, or toasted nuts. Adjust the amounts of the ingredients to suit your preferences.

13. Lentil soup with carrots and celery

Ingredients:
- 1 cup dry brown or green lentils, rinsed
- 4 cups low-sodium vegetable or chicken broth
- 2 tablespoons olive oil
- 1 onion, diced
- 3 carrots, peeled and diced
- 2 celery stalks, diced
- 3 garlic cloves, minced
- 1 teaspoon ground cumin
- 1 teaspoon dried thyme
- 1/4 teaspoon red pepper flakes (optional)
- Salt and pepper to taste
- Chopped parsley for garnish (optional)

Instructions:
1. In a large pot, combine the rinsed lentils and broth. Bring to a boil over high heat.

2. Reduce the heat to medium-low, cover, and simmer for 15-20 minutes, or until the lentils are tender.

3. In a separate skillet, heat the olive oil over medium heat. Add the onion, carrots, and celery. Sauté for 5-7 minutes, until the vegetables are softened.

4. Add the garlic, cumin, thyme, and red pepper flakes (if using) to the skillet. Cook for 1 minute, until fragrant.

5. Transfer the sautéed vegetables to the pot with the cooked lentils. Stir to combine.

6. Season the soup with salt and pepper to taste.

7. Simmer the soup for an additional 10-15 minutes to allow the flavors to meld.

8. Serve the lentil soup hot, garnished with chopped parsley if desired.

This lentil soup is packed with fiber, protein, and nutrients from the lentils, carrots, and celery. The cumin and thyme add warmth and depth of flavor. Adjust the seasoning to your liking.

Enjoy this comforting and nourishing lentil soup as a main dish or side. It's a great option for a healthy and satisfying meal.

14. Whole grain wrap with hummus, cucumber, and bell peppers

Ingredients:
- 1 whole grain tortilla or wrap
- 2-3 tablespoons hummus
- 1/4 cup sliced cucumber
- 1/4 cup sliced bell peppers (any color)
- 1-2 leaves of lettuce or spinach (optional)
- Salt and pepper to taste

Instructions:
1. Lay the whole grain tortilla or wrap on a flat surface.

2. Spread the hummus evenly over the center of the wrap, leaving a small border around the edges.

3. Arrange the sliced cucumber and bell peppers in a line down the center of the wrap.

4. If using, place the lettuce or spinach leaves on top of the vegetables.

5. Season with a pinch of salt and pepper.

6. Fold the bottom of the wrap up over the filling, then fold in the sides and continue rolling tightly into a wrap.

You can enjoy the wrap as is, or you can slice it in half diagonally to make it easier to eat.

Some variations and additions:
- Use different types of hummus, such as roasted red pepper or garlic hummus.
- Add other vegetables like shredded carrots, sprouts, or tomatoes.
- Include a protein source like grilled chicken, roasted chickpeas, or crumbled feta cheese.
- Drizzle with a bit of olive oil or balsamic vinegar.

This whole grain wrap makes for a quick, healthy, and portable lunch or snack. The combination of the creamy hummus, crunchy vegetables, and whole grain wrap is both satisfying and nutritious.

15. Brown rice and black bean burrito bowl

Ingredients:
- 1 cup uncooked brown rice
- 1 (15 oz) can black beans, rinsed and drained
- 1 cup diced tomatoes
- 1/2 cup diced onion
- 1 clove garlic, minced
- 1 teaspoon ground cumin
- 1/2 teaspoon chili powder
- Salt and pepper to taste
- Toppings (such as avocado, shredded cheese, salsa, cilantro, etc.)

Instructions:
1. Cook the brown rice according to package instructions.

2. In a medium saucepan, combine the rinsed and drained black beans, diced tomatoes, onion, garlic, cumin, and chili powder. Season with salt and pepper.

3. Heat the black bean mixture over medium heat, stirring occasionally, until heated through, about 5-7 minutes.

4. To assemble the burrito bowls, divide the cooked brown rice evenly among serving bowls.
5. Top the rice with the warm black bean mixture.

6. Add your desired toppings, such as diced avocado, shredded cheese, salsa, and chopped cilantro.

That's it! This burrito bowl is a delicious and nutritious meal that's easy to prepare.

Some variations:
- Use different types of beans, such as pinto or kidney beans.
- Add sautéed bell peppers or corn.
- Serve with a dollop of plain Greek yogurt or sour cream.
- Sprinkle toasted pepitas (pumpkin seeds) on top for extra crunch.

The combination of the nutty brown rice, flavorful black beans, and fresh toppings makes for a satisfying and well-balanced meal. Enjoy!

16. Spinach and chickpea salad with lemon dressing

Ingredients:
Salad:
- 5 oz baby spinach
- 1 (15 oz) can chickpeas, rinsed and drained
- 1 cup cherry tomatoes, halved
- 1/2 cup diced cucumber
- 1/4 cup crumbled feta cheese (optional)

Lemon Dressing:
- 2 tablespoons olive oil
- 2 tablespoons lemon juice
- 1 teaspoon Dijon mustard
- 1 teaspoon honey
- Salt and pepper to taste

Instructions:
1. In a large salad bowl, combine the baby spinach, chickpeas, cherry tomatoes, and diced cucumber.

2. In a small bowl, whisk together the olive oil, lemon juice, Dijon mustard, and honey. Season the dressing with salt and pepper to taste.

3. Drizzle the lemon dressing over the salad and toss gently to coat.

4. If using, sprinkle the crumbled feta cheese over the top of the salad.

That's it! This spinach and chickpea salad is a simple, yet flavorful and nutritious dish.

Some variations and additions:
- Add sliced avocado or roasted red peppers for extra flavor and texture.
- Sprinkle toasted nuts or seeds, such as almonds or sunflower seeds, for crunch.
- Use a different type of cheese, such as goat cheese or shredded cheddar.
- Toss in some cooked quinoa or bulgur for extra protein and fiber.

The lemon dressing provides a bright, tangy contrast to the earthy chickpeas and fresh spinach. This salad makes for a great lunch or light dinner option. Enjoy!

17. Quinoa salad with roasted vegetables and feta cheese

Ingredients:
- 1 cup uncooked quinoa, rinsed
- 2 cups vegetable or chicken broth
- 1 medium zucchini, diced
- 1 red bell pepper, diced
- 1 cup cherry tomatoes, halved
- 1/2 red onion, diced
- 2 tablespoons olive oil
- Salt and pepper to taste
- 1/2 cup crumbled feta cheese
- 2 tablespoons chopped fresh parsley

Dressing:
- 2 tablespoons olive oil
- 2 tablespoons lemon juice
- 1 teaspoon Dijon mustard
- 1 teaspoon honey
- Salt and pepper to taste

Instructions:

1. Preheat your oven to 400°F (200°C).

2. In a medium saucepan, combine the rinsed quinoa and broth. Bring to a boil, then reduce heat, cover, and simmer for 15-20 minutes, until the quinoa is cooked and fluffy. Fluff with a fork and set aside to cool.

3. On a large baking sheet, toss the diced zucchini, bell pepper, cherry tomatoes, and red onion with the 2 tablespoons of olive oil. Season with salt and pepper.

4. Roast the vegetables in the preheated oven for 20-25 minutes, stirring halfway, until they are tender and lightly caramelized.

5. In a large bowl, combine the cooked quinoa, roasted vegetables, crumbled feta cheese, and chopped parsley.

6. In a small bowl, whisk together the dressing ingredients: the 2 tablespoons of olive oil, lemon juice, Dijon mustard, honey, and salt and pepper to taste. Drizzle the dressing over the quinoa salad and toss gently to coat.

Serve the quinoa salad warm or chilled. The combination of the fluffy quinoa, roasted vegetables, tangy feta, and bright dressing makes for a delicious and nutritious meal or side dish.

18. Smoked salmon with avocado and whole grain toast

Ingredients:
- 2 slices of whole grain bread
- 1 ripe avocado, mashed
- 4 oz smoked salmon
- 1 tablespoon lemon juice
- 1 teaspoon capers (optional)
- Salt and pepper to taste
- Chopped fresh dill for garnish (optional)

Instructions:
1. Toast the whole grain bread until lightly golden.

2. In a small bowl, mash the avocado with the lemon juice. Season with a pinch of salt and pepper.

3. Spread the mashed avocado evenly over the toasted bread slices.

4. Top the avocado toast with slices of smoked salmon.

5. If using, sprinkle the capers over the salmon.

6. Garnish with chopped fresh dill, if desired.

That's it! This smoked salmon and avocado toast makes for a simple, yet delicious and nutritious breakfast or snack.

Some variations and tips:
- Use a different type of bread, such as sourdough or rye, if preferred.
- Add a drizzle of olive oil or a sprinkle of everything bagel seasoning for extra flavor.
- Swap the smoked salmon for canned tuna or grilled chicken for a different protein option.
- Serve the avocado toast with a side of mixed greens or a hard-boiled egg for a more substantial meal.

The healthy fats from the avocado and salmon, combined with the fiber and nutrients from the whole grain bread, make this a nutritious and satisfying breakfast or snack. Enjoy!

19. Turkey and spinach whole grain sandwich

Ingredients:
- 2 slices of whole grain bread
- 2-3 ounces sliced turkey breast
- 1 cup fresh spinach leaves
- 1 slice of tomato (optional)
- 1 tablespoon hummus or avocado spread (optional)
- Salt and pepper to taste

Instructions:
1. Lay the two slices of whole grain bread on a clean surface.

2. Spread the hummus or avocado spread (if using) evenly on one slice of bread.

3. Layer the sliced turkey breast on top of the hummus or avocado.

4. Top the turkey with the fresh spinach leaves.

5. If using, place the slice of tomato on top of the spinach.

6. Season the sandwich with a pinch of salt and pepper.

7. Place the remaining slice of bread on top to complete the sandwich.

That's it! This turkey and spinach whole grain sandwich is a simple, yet nutritious and satisfying option for lunch or a snack.

Some variations and additions:

- Use different types of whole grain bread, such as whole wheat, rye, or multigrain.

- Add other vegetables like sliced cucumber, bell peppers, or sprouts.

- Swap the turkey for grilled chicken, tuna salad, or roasted vegetables.

- Include a slice of cheese, such as cheddar or provolone.

- Drizzle a bit of olive oil or balsamic vinegar over the spinach.

The combination of the lean protein from the turkey, the fiber and nutrients from the whole grain bread and spinach, and the optional healthy fats from the hummus or avocado make this a well-balanced and satisfying sandwich. Enjoy!

20. Sweet potato and black bean salad

Ingredients:
- 2 tablespoons chopped fresh cilantro
- 2 tablespoons olive oil
- 2 tablespoons lime juice
- 1 teaspoon ground cumin
- 1/4 teaspoon chili powder
- Salt and pepper to taste
- 2 medium sweet potatoes, peeled and diced
- 1 (15 oz) can black beans, rinsed and drained
- 1 red bell pepper, diced
- 1/2 red onion, diced
- 1 cup cherry tomatoes, halved

Instructions:
1. Preheat your oven to 400°F (200°C).

2. Spread the diced sweet potatoes on a baking sheet and toss with 1 tablespoon of the olive oil. Season with a pinch of salt and pepper.

3. Roast the sweet potatoes in the preheated oven for 20-25 minutes, or until they are tender and lightly browned. Allow to cool slightly.

4. In a large bowl, combine the roasted sweet potatoes, black beans, diced bell pepper, red onion, and cherry tomatoes.

5. In a small bowl, whisk together the remaining 1 tablespoon of olive oil, lime juice, cumin, and chili powder. Season the dressing with salt and pepper to taste.

6. Pour the dressing over the salad and toss gently to coat. Sprinkle the chopped fresh cilantro over the top of the salad.

Serve the sweet potato and black bean salad at room temperature or chilled. This salad makes a great side dish or a light main course.

Variations and additions:
- Add diced avocado for extra creaminess.
- Sprinkle crumbled feta or queso fresco over the top.
- Toss in some cooked quinoa or brown rice for extra protein and fiber.
- Use a different type of bean, such as pinto or kidney beans.

The combination of the sweet roasted potatoes, earthy black beans, and bright, tangy dressing makes for a delicious and nutritious salad. Enjoy!

21. Greek salad with a side of whole grain pita

Ingredients:
Greek Salad:
- 5 oz mixed greens (such as romaine, spinach, and arugula)
- 1 cup cherry tomatoes, halved
- 1/2 cucumber, diced
- 1/4 red onion, thinly sliced
- 1/2 cup pitted kalamata olives, halved
- 1/2 cup crumbled feta cheese
- 2 tablespoons olive oil
- 1 tablespoon red wine vinegar
- 1 teaspoon dried oregano
- Salt and pepper to taste

Whole Grain Pita:
- 2 whole grain pita breads

Instructions:

1. In a large salad bowl, combine the mixed greens, cherry tomatoes, cucumber, red onion, kalamata olives, and crumbled feta cheese.

2. In a small bowl, whisk together the olive oil, red wine vinegar, and dried oregano. Season the dressing with salt and pepper to taste.

3. Drizzle the dressing over the salad and toss gently to coat.

4. Serve the Greek salad with the whole grain pita breads on the side.

To serve, you can either tear the pita bread into pieces and use it to scoop up the salad, or slice the pita into wedges to enjoy alongside the salad.

Variations and additions:
- Add grilled chicken or chickpeas for extra protein.
- Include diced bell peppers or artichoke hearts.
- Swap the feta for crumbled goat cheese or shredded mozzarella.
- Drizzle the salad with a bit of lemon juice or balsamic glaze.

The combination of the fresh, crunchy vegetables, tangy feta, and flavorful Greek dressing makes for a delicious and nutritious salad. The whole grain pita provides a satisfying and fiber-rich accompaniment.

22. Tofu stir-fry with broccoli and bell peppers

Ingredients:
- 2 tablespoons low-sodium soy sauce
- 1 tablespoon rice vinegar
- 1 teaspoon honey
- 1/4 teaspoon red pepper flakes (optional)
- Salt and pepper to taste
- Cooked brown rice, for serving
- 1 block (14 oz) extra-firm tofu, pressed and cubed
- 2 tablespoons sesame oil
- 2 cups broccoli florets
- 1 red bell pepper, sliced
- 1 yellow bell pepper, sliced
- 3 cloves garlic, minced
- 1 tablespoon grated fresh ginger

Instructions:

1. In a large skillet or wok, heat the sesame oil over medium-high heat.

2. Add the cubed tofu and cook, stirring occasionally, until lightly browned on all sides, about 5-7 minutes. Transfer the tofu to a plate and set aside.

3. In the same skillet, add the broccoli florets and bell pepper slices. Stir-fry for 3-4 minutes, until the vegetables are starting to soften.

4. Add the minced garlic and grated ginger to the skillet. Cook for 1 minute, until fragrant.

5. Return the cooked tofu to the skillet. Add the soy sauce, rice vinegar, honey, and red pepper flakes (if using). Stir to combine.

6. Cook the stir-fry for an additional 2-3 minutes, until the vegetables are tender and the sauce has thickened slightly.

7. Season the stir-fry with salt and pepper to taste. Serve the tofu and vegetable stir-fry over cooked brown rice.

This tofu stir-fry is a delicious and nutritious meatless meal. The combination of the firm tofu, crunchy vegetables, and savory-sweet sauce is both satisfying and flavorful.

Variations and tips:
- Use a different protein, such as chicken or shrimp, instead of tofu.
- Swap the vegetables for your favorites, such as snow peas, mushrooms, or bok choy.
- Serve the stir-fry over quinoa or cauliflower rice for a low-carb option.
- Top with toasted sesame seeds or sliced green onions for extra flavor and texture.

23. Baked salmon with asparagus and quinoa

Ingredients:
- 4 (6 oz) salmon fillets
- 1 lb asparagus, trimmed
- 1 cup uncooked quinoa, rinsed
- 2 cups low-sodium chicken or vegetable broth
- 2 tablespoons olive oil, divided
- 1 teaspoon lemon zest
- 2 tablespoons lemon juice
- 2 cloves garlic, minced
- 1 teaspoon dried dill
- Salt and pepper to taste

Instructions:
1. Preheat your oven to 400°F (200°C).

2. In a medium saucepan, combine the rinsed quinoa and broth. Bring to a boil, then reduce heat, cover, and simmer for 15-20 minutes, until the quinoa is cooked and fluffy. Fluff with a fork and set aside.

3. Arrange the salmon fillets and asparagus spears on a large baking sheet. Drizzle with 1 tablespoon of the olive oil and season with salt and pepper.

4. In a small bowl, mix together the remaining 1 tablespoon of olive oil, lemon zest, lemon juice, garlic, and dried dill. Pour this mixture over the salmon and asparagus, making sure to coat everything evenly.

5. Bake the salmon and asparagus in the preheated oven for 12-15 minutes, or until the salmon is cooked through and the asparagus is tender. Serve the baked salmon and asparagus over the cooked quinoa.

This baked salmon dish is a complete and nutritious meal, with the salmon providing healthy omega-3 fatty acids, the asparagus offering fiber and vitamins, and the quinoa contributing complex carbs and protein.

Variations and tips:
- Use different types of fish, such as trout or halibut, instead of salmon.
- Swap the asparagus for other roasted vegetables, like Brussels sprouts or sweet potatoes.
- Add a sprinkle of grated Parmesan cheese or chopped fresh herbs on top.
- Serve with a side salad or a dollop of Greek yogurt for extra creaminess.

24. Grilled chicken with sweet potatoes and green beans

Ingredients:
- 4 boneless, skinless chicken breasts
- 2 medium sweet potatoes, peeled and cubed
- 1 lb green beans, trimmed
- 2 tablespoons olive oil, divided
- 1 teaspoon garlic powder
- 1 teaspoon paprika
- Salt and pepper to taste

Instructions:
1. Preheat your grill or grill pan to medium-high heat.

2. In a large bowl, toss the cubed sweet potatoes with 1 tablespoon of the olive oil, garlic powder, and a pinch of salt and pepper.

3. Spread the seasoned sweet potato cubes on a baking sheet and roast in the oven at 400°F (200°C) for 20-25 minutes, or until tender and lightly browned.

4. In another bowl, toss the trimmed green beans with the remaining 1 tablespoon of olive oil and season with salt and pepper.

5. Grill the chicken breasts for 5-7 minutes per side, or until cooked through. Transfer the grilled chicken to a plate and let it rest for a few minutes.

6. Add the seasoned green beans to the grill and cook for 5-7 minutes, turning occasionally, until tender-crisp. Serve the grilled chicken alongside the roasted sweet potatoes and grilled green beans.

This grilled chicken with sweet potatoes and green beans is a well-balanced and nutritious meal. The sweet potatoes provide complex carbohydrates and fiber, while the green beans offer vitamins and minerals. The grilled chicken is a lean protein source.

Variations and tips:
- Marinate the chicken in a mixture of olive oil, lemon juice, and herbs before grilling.
- Roast the sweet potatoes and green beans together on the same baking sheet for easier preparation.
- Add a sprinkle of grated Parmesan cheese or chopped fresh herbs to the vegetables.
- Serve with a side of quinoa or brown rice for extra fiber and protein.

25. Vegetable stir-fry with tofu and brown rice

Ingredients:
- 1 cup uncooked brown rice
- 1 block (14 oz) extra-firm tofu, pressed and cubed
- 2 tablespoons sesame oil, divided
- 2 cups broccoli florets
- 1 red bell pepper, sliced
- 1 cup sliced mushrooms
- 1 cup snow peas
- 3 cloves garlic, minced
- 1 tablespoon grated fresh ginger
- 2 tablespoons low-sodium soy sauce
- 1 tablespoon rice vinegar
- 1 teaspoon honey
- Salt and pepper to taste
- Chopped green onions and sesame seeds for garnish (optional)

Instructions:

1. Cook the brown rice according to package instructions. Set aside. In a large skillet or wok, heat 1 tablespoon of the sesame oil over medium-high heat.

2. Add the cubed tofu and cook, stirring occasionally, until lightly browned on all sides, about 5-7 minutes. Transfer the tofu to a plate and set aside. In the same skillet, heat the remaining 1 tablespoon of sesame oil.

3. Add the broccoli florets, bell pepper slices, mushrooms, and snow peas. Stir-fry for 4-5 minutes, until the vegetables are tender-crisp. Add the minced garlic and grated ginger to the skillet. Cook for 1 minute, until fragrant.

4. Return the cooked tofu to the skillet. Add the soy sauce, rice vinegar, and honey. Stir to combine.

5. Cook the stir-fry for an additional 2-3 minutes, until the sauce has thickened slightly. Season the stir-fry with salt and pepper to taste.

6. Serve the vegetable and tofu stir-fry over the cooked brown rice. Garnish with chopped green onions and sesame seeds, if desired.

This vegetable stir-fry with tofu and brown rice is a nutritious and flavorful meatless meal. The combination of the firm tofu, crunchy vegetables, and savory-sweet sauce is both satisfying and delicious.

Variations and tips:
- Use a different protein, such as chicken or shrimp, instead of tofu.
- Swap the vegetables for your favorites, such as bok choy, carrots, or zucchini.
- Serve the stir-fry over quinoa or cauliflower rice for a low-carb option.
- Add a splash of sriracha or chili oil for a spicy kick.

26. Beef and vegetable stew with barley

Ingredients:
- 1 lb (450g) beef stew meat, cubed
- 1 cup pearl barley, rinsed
- 4 cups beef broth
- 2 cups water
- 2 tablespoons olive oil
- 1 onion, diced
- 2 carrots, peeled and diced
- 2 celery stalks, diced
- 3 cloves garlic, minced
- 2 bay leaves
- 1 teaspoon dried thyme
- Salt and pepper to taste
- Chopped fresh parsley for garnish (optional)

Instructions:
1. Heat the olive oil in a large pot or Dutch oven over medium heat. Add the beef cubes and brown them on all sides, about 5-7 minutes. Remove the beef from the pot and set aside.

2. In the same pot, add a little more oil if needed, then add the diced onions, carrots, and celery. Cook until the vegetables are softened, about 5 minutes.

3. Add the minced garlic to the pot and cook for an additional minute until fragrant.

4. Return the browned beef to the pot. Add the rinsed barley, beef broth, water, bay leaves, and dried thyme. Stir well to combine.

5. Bring the stew to a boil, then reduce the heat to low. Cover the pot and let the stew simmer for about 1 to 1.5 hours, or until the beef is tender and the barley is cooked through. Stir occasionally and add more water if needed to reach your desired consistency.

6. Once the stew is ready, season with salt and pepper to taste. Remove the bay leaves before serving.

7. Ladle the beef and vegetable stew into bowls and garnish with chopped fresh parsley if desired. Serve hot and enjoy!

This stew is even better the next day as the flavors have had time to meld together, so don't hesitate to make extra for leftovers!

27. Baked cod with a side of roasted Brussels sprouts

Ingredients:
- 4 cod fillets (6 oz each)
- 1 lemon (zested and juiced)
- 3 cloves garlic, minced
- 1 tsp dried thyme
- 1 tsp paprika
- Salt and pepper
- Fresh parsley
- 1 lb Brussels sprouts, halved
- 2 tbsp olive oil
- 1 tsp garlic powder
- 1 tbsp balsamic vinegar (optional)

Instructions:

1. Preheat oven to 400°F (200°C).

2. Toss Brussels sprouts with olive oil, garlic powder, salt, and pepper. Roast for 20-25 mins.

3. Combine olive oil, lemon zest, lemon juice, minced garlic, thyme, paprika, salt, and pepper. Brush over cod fillets.

4. Bake cod at 375°F (190°C) for 12-15 mins until opaque and flaky.

5. Garnish cod with parsley. Drizzle Brussels sprouts with balsamic vinegar (optional).

6. Serve cod with roasted Brussels sprouts. Enjoy!

28. Whole grain spaghetti with turkey meatballs

Ingredients:
For Turkey Meatballs:
- 1 lb ground turkey
- 1/2 cup breadcrumbs (whole grain, if available)
- 1/4 cup grated Parmesan cheese
- 1 egg
- 2 cloves garlic, minced
- 1 teaspoon dried oregano
- 1 teaspoon dried basil
- Salt and pepper to taste
- Olive oil for cooking

For Whole Grain Spaghetti:
- 8 oz whole grain spaghetti
- Salt for pasta water

For Serving:
- Marinara sauce
- Fresh basil leaves (optional)
- Grated Parmesan cheese (optional)

Instructions:
1. Preheat the oven to 400°F (200°C).

2. In a large mixing bowl, combine ground turkey, breadcrumbs, grated Parmesan cheese, egg, minced garlic, dried oregano, dried basil, salt, and pepper. Mix until well combined.

3. Form the mixture into meatballs, about 1 inch in diameter.

4. Heat olive oil in a large skillet over medium heat. Add the meatballs and cook until browned on all sides, about 8-10 minutes.

5. Transfer the browned meatballs to a baking sheet lined with parchment paper and bake in the preheated oven for 10-12 minutes, or until cooked through.

6. While the meatballs are baking, cook the whole grain spaghetti according to the package instructions in salted water until al dente.

7. Once the spaghetti is cooked, drain it and return it to the pot. Toss the spaghetti with marinara sauce until well coated.

8. Serve the whole grain spaghetti topped with turkey meatballs. Garnish with fresh basil leaves and grated Parmesan cheese if desired.

Enjoy your wholesome and delicious whole grain spaghetti with turkey meatballs!

29. Chicken curry with brown rice

Ingredients:
- 1 lb boneless, skinless chicken
- 1 onion, chopped
- 2 cloves garlic, minced
- 1 tbsp ginger, minced
- 2 tbsp curry powder
- 1 tsp each ground turmeric, cumin, and coriander
- 1 can (14 oz) coconut milk
- 1 cup chicken broth
- 2 tbsp tomato paste
- 2 tbsp olive oil
- Salt and pepper
- Fresh cilantro (optional)

For Brown Rice:
- 1 cup brown rice
- 2 cups water
- Salt

Instructions:

1. Cook brown rice according to package instructions.

2. Sauté onion, garlic, and ginger in olive oil until softened.

3. Add chicken, spices, coconut milk, broth, and tomato paste. Simmer for 20-25 mins.

4. Season with salt and pepper.

5. Serve curry over brown rice.

6. Garnish with cilantro if desired.

Enjoy your Chicken Curry with Brown Rice!

30. Quinoa-stuffed bell peppers

Ingredients:
- 4 large bell peppers, any color
- 1 cup quinoa, rinsed
- 2 cups vegetable broth or water
- 1 tablespoon olive oil
- 1 onion, diced
- 2 cloves garlic, minced
- 1 zucchini, diced
- 1 carrot, diced
- 1 cup diced tomatoes (fresh or canned)
- 1 teaspoon dried oregano
- 1 teaspoon dried basil
- Salt and pepper to taste
- 1 cup shredded cheese (cheddar, mozzarella, or your choice)
- Fresh parsley or cilantro for garnish (optional)

Instructions:
1. Preheat your oven to 375°F (190°C).

2. Cut the tops off the bell peppers and remove the seeds and membranes. Set aside.

3. In a medium saucepan, combine the quinoa and vegetable broth or water. Bring to a boil, then reduce the heat to low, cover, and simmer for about 15 minutes, or until the quinoa is cooked and fluffy. Remove from heat and set aside.

4. In a large skillet, heat olive oil over medium heat. Add diced onion and cook until translucent, about 3-4 minutes. Add minced garlic and cook for an additional minute.

5. Add diced zucchini and carrot to the skillet. Cook for about 5 minutes, or until the vegetables are tender.

6. Stir in the diced tomatoes, dried oregano, dried basil, cooked quinoa, salt, and pepper. Cook for another 2-3 minutes to allow the flavors to meld together. Taste and adjust seasoning if needed.

7. Place the hollowed-out bell peppers in a baking dish. Fill each pepper with the quinoa and vegetable mixture, pressing down gently to pack it in.

8. Sprinkle shredded cheese over the top of each stuffed pepper.

9. Cover the baking dish with aluminum foil and bake in the preheated oven for 25-30 minutes, or until the peppers are tender and the cheese is melted and bubbly.

10. Remove from the oven and let the stuffed peppers cool for a few minutes before serving. Garnish with fresh parsley or cilantro if desired, and serve hot.

31. Shrimp and vegetable kebabs with a side of farro

Ingredients:
For Shrimp and Vegetable Kebabs:
- 1 lb large shrimp, peeled and deveined
- 2 bell peppers, cut into chunks
- 1 zucchini, sliced
- 1 red onion, cut into chunks
- 8-10 cherry tomatoes
- Wooden or metal skewers
(if using wooden skewers, soak them
 in water for 30 minutes to prevent burning)
- Olive oil for brushing
- Salt and pepper to taste
- Lemon wedges for serving
- Fresh parsley for garnish (optional)

For Farro:
- 1 cup farro
- 3 cups water or vegetable broth
- Salt to taste
- 1 tablespoon olive oil (optional)

Instructions:
For Farro:
1. Rinse the farro under cold water.
2. In a medium saucepan, combine the rinsed farro and water or vegetable broth. Add a pinch of salt.
3. Bring to a boil, then reduce the heat to low, cover, and simmer for about 25-30 minutes, or until the farro is tender but still chewy.
4. Drain any excess liquid and fluff the farro with a fork. If desired, stir in olive oil for extra flavor. Set aside.

For Shrimp and Vegetable Kebabs:
1. Preheat your grill or grill pan over medium-high heat.

2. Thread the shrimp, bell peppers, zucchini, red onion, and cherry tomatoes onto skewers, alternating between each ingredient. Season the kebabs with salt and pepper.

3. Brush the assembled kebabs with olive oil to prevent sticking.

4. Place the kebabs on the preheated grill and cook for 2-3 minutes per side, or until the shrimp are pink and opaque and the vegetables are charred and tender.

5. Remove the kebabs from the grill and transfer them to a serving platter. Serve the shrimp and vegetable kebabs hot with cooked farro on the side. Garnish with fresh parsley and lemon wedges for squeezing over the kebabs before serving.

32. Grilled pork chops with a kale and apple salad

For Grilled Pork Chops:
- 4 pork chops
- 2 tbsp olive oil
- 2 cloves garlic, minced
- 1 tsp dried thyme
- 1 tsp paprika
- Salt and pepper

For Kale & Apple Salad:
- 4 cups kale, chopped
- 1 apple, thinly sliced
- 1/4 cup chopped walnuts or almonds
- 1/4 cup dried cranberries or raisins
- 2 tbsp lemon juice
- 2 tbsp olive oil
- 1 tbsp honey or maple syrup
- Salt and pepper

Instructions:

1. Preheat grill to medium-high heat.

2. Rub pork chops with olive oil, garlic, thyme, paprika, salt, and pepper.

3. Grill pork chops for 4-5 mins per side until cooked through.

4. For the salad, combine kale, apple, nuts, and dried fruit in a bowl.

5. Whisk lemon juice, olive oil, honey, salt, and pepper for dressing.

6. Toss salad with dressing.

7. Serve grilled pork chops with kale & apple salad.

Enjoy your meal!

33. Eggplant Parmesan with whole wheat pasta

Ingredients:
- 1 large eggplant, sliced into 1/2-inch thick rounds
- 1 cup whole wheat breadcrumbs
- 1/2 cup grated Parmesan cheese
- 2 eggs, beaten
- 2 cups marinara sauce
- 8 oz whole wheat pasta
- 1 cup shredded mozzarella cheese

Instructions:
1. Preheat oven to 375°F. Line a baking sheet with parchment paper.

2. In a shallow bowl, combine the breadcrumbs and Parmesan cheese. In another shallow bowl, place the beaten eggs.

3. Dip the eggplant slices into the egg, then coat both sides with the breadcrumb mixture. Place the breaded eggplant slices in a single layer on the prepared baking sheet.

4. Bake for 20-25 minutes, flipping halfway, until the eggplant is tender and golden brown.

5. Meanwhile, cook the whole wheat pasta according to package instructions. Drain and set aside.

6. In a baking dish, layer half the eggplant slices on the bottom. Top with 1 cup of the marinara sauce and half the mozzarella cheese. Repeat the layers.

7. Bake for 20-25 minutes, until the cheese is melted and bubbly.

8. Serve the eggplant Parmesan over the cooked whole wheat pasta. Enjoy!

34. Apple slices with almond butter

Ingredients:
- 2 medium apples, cored and sliced
- 1/4 cup creamy almond butter

Instructions:

1. Wash and core the apples. Slice them into thin, even slices.

2. Arrange the apple slices on a plate or platter.

3. Scoop the almond butter into a small bowl or ramekin.

4. Serve the apple slices alongside the almond butter for dipping.

That's it! This makes a quick, healthy, and delicious snack or light dessert. The creamy almond butter pairs perfectly with the crisp, sweet apple slices.

You can use any variety of apple you prefer. Some good options are Gala, Fuji, Honeycrisp, or Pink Lady.

For extra flavor, you can sprinkle a pinch of cinnamon over the apple slices before serving. You can also try using peanut butter or another nut butter instead of almond butter if you prefer.

This is a simple, nutritious, and satisfying snack that takes just minutes to prepare. Enjoy!

35. Carrot sticks with hummus

Ingredients:
- 4-5 medium carrots, peeled and cut into sticks
- 1 cup prepared hummus

Instructions:

1. Wash and peel the carrots. Cut them into long, thin sticks, about 4-5 inches long and 1/2 inch thick.

2. Place the carrot sticks in a bowl or on a plate.

3. Scoop the hummus into a small serving bowl or ramekin.

4. Arrange the carrot sticks around the hummus, making it easy to dip them.

That's it! This simple snack is healthy, flavorful, and satisfying.

The crunchy, sweet carrot sticks pair perfectly with the creamy, savory hummus. Hummus is a great source of protein, fiber, and healthy fats from the chickpeas and tahini.

You can use any variety of carrot you prefer - baby carrots, rainbow carrots, or regular orange carrots all work well.

For extra flavor, you can try different hummus varieties like roasted red pepper, garlic, or Mediterranean herb. You can also sprinkle a bit of paprika, cumin, or za'atar over the hummus.

This makes a great snack, appetizer, or healthy side dish. It's easy to prepare and perfect for dipping. Enjoy!

36. Mixed nuts and seeds

Ingredients:
- 1/2 cup raw almonds
- 1/2 cup raw cashews
- 1/4 cup raw pumpkin seeds (pepitas)
- 1/4 cup raw sunflower seeds
- 1/4 cup raw walnuts
- 1/4 cup raw pecans
- 1 tsp ground cinnamon (optional)
- 1/4 tsp sea salt (optional)

Instructions:

1. In a medium bowl, combine all the nuts and seeds.

2. If desired, sprinkle the cinnamon and sea salt over the nut and seed mixture and stir to coat evenly.

3. Transfer the mixed nuts and seeds to an airtight container or resealable bag.

That's it! This makes a delicious, nutritious snack that you can enjoy on its own or use as a topping for yogurt, oatmeal, or salads.

The combination of different nuts and seeds provides a variety of healthy fats, proteins, fiber, vitamins, and minerals. Some great options to include are:

- Almonds - rich in healthy fats, protein, and fiber
- Cashews - creamy and packed with nutrients
- Pumpkin seeds - a good source of magnesium and zinc
- Sunflower seeds - high in vitamin E and antioxidants
- Walnuts - contain anti-inflammatory omega-3s
- Pecans - provide beneficial plant compounds

You can adjust the amounts and types of nuts and seeds to your personal preference. The cinnamon and salt are optional but add a nice flavor boost.

Store the mixed nuts and seeds in an airtight container at room temperature for up to 2 weeks. Enjoy as a healthy snack anytime!

37. Greek yogurt with granola

Ingredients:
- 1 cup plain Greek yogurt
- 1/2 cup granola
- 1 tbsp honey (optional)
- Fresh fruit (such as berries, sliced banana, or diced mango), for topping (optional)

Instructions:

1. Scoop the Greek yogurt into a bowl or parfait glass.

2. Sprinkle the granola evenly over the top of the yogurt.

3. If desired, drizzle the honey over the granola.

4. Top with any fresh fruit you'd like, such as berries, sliced banana, or diced mango.

That's it! This simple, nutritious parfait makes a great breakfast, snack, or healthy dessert.

The creamy Greek yogurt provides protein, calcium, and probiotics. The granola adds a satisfying crunch and complex carbohydrates. The honey and fruit provide natural sweetness.

You can use any type of plain Greek yogurt you prefer - full-fat, low-fat, or non-fat. For the granola, choose a store-bought variety or make your own homemade granola.

Feel free to adjust the amounts of each ingredient to your taste. You can use more or less yogurt, granola, honey, and fruit as desired.

This is a versatile and customizable recipe that's easy to prepare. It's a delicious and nutritious way to start your day or enjoy a healthy snack. Enjoy!

38. Fresh fruit salad

Ingredients:
- 1 cup diced pineapple
- 1 cup diced mango
- 1 cup halved strawberries
- 1 cup blueberries
- 1 cup diced kiwi
- 1 tbsp fresh lemon juice
- 1 tbsp honey (optional)

Instructions:

1. In a large bowl, combine the diced pineapple, mango, strawberries, blueberries, and kiwi.

2. Drizzle the lemon juice over the fruit and gently toss to coat.

3. If desired, drizzle the honey over the fruit salad and toss again to combine.

4. Cover and refrigerate for at least 30 minutes to allow the flavors to meld.

5. Serve chilled.

That's it! This fresh fruit salad is a delicious and nutritious snack or dessert.

The combination of pineapple, mango, strawberries, blueberries, and kiwi provides a variety of vitamins, minerals, and antioxidants. The lemon juice adds a bright, refreshing flavor.

You can use any combination of fresh, seasonal fruits that you enjoy. Other great options include:

- Diced apples or pears
- Halved grapes
- Cubed watermelon or cantaloupe
- Sliced bananas
- Chopped peaches or nectarines

The honey is optional, but it can add a nice touch of sweetness if the fruit isn't quite ripe enough.

This fruit salad is best enjoyed within 2-3 days of making it. Store it covered in the refrigerator. Enjoy this colorful, healthy treat!

39. Cottage cheese with pineapple chunks

Ingredients:
- 1 cup low-fat or non-fat cottage cheese
- 1/2 cup diced fresh pineapple chunks
- 1 tsp honey (optional)

Instructions:

1. Scoop the cottage cheese into a bowl or serving dish.

2. Top the cottage cheese with the diced pineapple chunks.

3. If desired, drizzle the honey over the top.

That's it! This makes a quick, easy, and nutritious snack or light meal.

The combination of creamy cottage cheese and sweet pineapple chunks is both delicious and satisfying. The cottage cheese provides protein, while the pineapple adds natural sweetness and vitamin C.

You can use any type of cottage cheese you prefer - low-fat, non-fat, or full-fat. The honey is optional, but it can add a nice touch of sweetness if the pineapple isn't quite ripe enough.

For extra flavor, you can also try adding:
- A sprinkle of cinnamon
- A drizzle of vanilla extract
- A handful of chopped nuts or granola

This is a versatile and customizable snack that takes just minutes to prepare. It's a great way to enjoy the refreshing taste of pineapple with the creaminess of cottage cheese. Enjoy!

40. Dark chocolate and almonds

Ingredients:
- 1 oz dark chocolate, chopped or broken into pieces
- 1/4 cup raw, unsalted almonds

Instructions:

1. Place the chopped dark chocolate in a small bowl.

2. Add the raw almonds to the bowl with the chocolate.

3. Enjoy the dark chocolate and almonds together as a snack.

That's it! This is a quick, easy, and nutritious snack that combines the rich flavor of dark chocolate with the crunch and healthy fats of almonds.

Some tips:

- Choose a high-quality dark chocolate with at least 70% cacao content for maximum health benefits.
- Use raw, unsalted almonds to avoid added oils or salt.
- Adjust the portion sizes to your liking - 1 oz of dark chocolate and 1/4 cup almonds is a good starting point.
- You can also try different nut varieties like cashews, pecans, or walnuts.

The dark chocolate provides antioxidants, while the almonds offer protein, fiber, and healthy monounsaturated fats. Together, they make a satisfying and nutrient-dense snack.

This is a great option when you're craving something sweet and indulgent, but still want a healthy treat. The combination of flavors and textures is simply delicious. Enjoy!

41. Edamame with sea salt

Ingredients:
- 1 lb frozen edamame in the pod
- 1 tsp sea salt

Instructions:

1. Bring a large pot of water to a boil.

2. Add the frozen edamame pods to the boiling water. Cook for 5-7 minutes, until the pods are bright green and tender.

3. Drain the edamame and transfer to a serving bowl.

4. Sprinkle the sea salt over the hot edamame and toss to coat evenly.

5. Serve the edamame warm, with the pods still intact.

That's it! This makes a quick, healthy, and delicious snack or appetizer.

Edamame are young, immature soybeans that are packed with protein, fiber, vitamins, and minerals. The sea salt adds a nice savory flavor that complements the natural sweetness of the edamame.

You can adjust the amount of salt to your taste preference. Some other seasoning ideas include:

- Garlic powder
- Chili powder or cayenne pepper
- Lemon or lime zest
- Toasted sesame seeds

Edamame are typically served in the pod, so guests can pop the beans directly from the pod into their mouths. Provide a small bowl for the empty pods.

This is a simple, nutritious snack that's easy to prepare. Enjoy the edamame warm, straight from the pot. Any leftovers can be stored in the refrigerator for 2-3 days.

42. Hard-boiled eggs

Ingredients:
- 6 large eggs

Instructions:

1. Place the eggs in a single layer in a saucepan and cover with cold water by 1 inch.

2. Bring the water to a boil over high heat. Once the water reaches a full boil, remove the pan from the heat and cover.

3. Let the eggs sit in the hot water for the following times:
   - For soft-boiled eggs: 6-7 minutes
   - For hard-boiled eggs: 12 minutes

4. Drain the hot water and cover the eggs with cold water to stop the cooking. Let sit for 5 minutes.

5. Peel the eggs and enjoy!

That's it! This method produces perfectly cooked hard-boiled eggs every time.

Some tips:

- Use eggs that are at least a week old, as they are easier to peel.
- Start with cold water to allow the eggs to come up to temperature gradually.
- The timing may need to be adjusted slightly based on the size of your eggs and your altitude.
- To peel, gently tap the egg all over on a hard surface, then roll between your hands to loosen the shell.

Hard-boiled eggs are a great source of protein, vitamins, and minerals. They make a convenient, portable snack or can be used in recipes like egg salad, deviled eggs, or as a topping for salads.

You can store peeled hard-boiled eggs in the refrigerator for up to 1 week. Enjoy your perfectly cooked hard-boiled eggs!

43. Smoothie with spinach, berries, and kefir

Ingredients:
- 1 cup fresh spinach leaves
- 1 cup frozen mixed berries (such as blueberries, raspberries, and blackberries)
- 1 cup plain kefir
- 1/2 banana, frozen
- 1 tbsp honey (optional)
- 1/4 cup water or milk of your choice (if needed to blend)

Instructions:

1. Add the spinach, frozen berries, kefir, and frozen banana to a high-powered blender.

2. Blend on high speed until the mixture is smooth and creamy, about 1-2 minutes.

3. If the smoothie is too thick, add 1-2 tablespoons of water or milk to thin it out.

4. If desired, drizzle in the honey and blend again briefly to incorporate.

5. Pour the smoothie into a glass and enjoy immediately.

This smoothie is packed with nutrients from the spinach, berries, and kefir. The spinach provides vitamins, minerals, and antioxidants, while the berries offer natural sweetness and more antioxidants. The kefir adds probiotics, protein, and creaminess.

The frozen banana helps thicken the smoothie and provides natural sweetness. The honey is optional, but can add an extra touch of sweetness if desired.

You can use any type of berries you like - strawberries, blueberries, raspberries, and blackberries all work well. Feel free to adjust the ingredient amounts to suit your taste preferences.

This makes a delicious, nutritious, and refreshing smoothie that's perfect for breakfast, a snack, or anytime you want a healthy boost. Enjoy!

44. Rice cakes with avocado and cherry tomatoes

Ingredients:
- 2 whole grain rice cakes
- 1/2 ripe avocado, mashed
- 8-10 cherry tomatoes, halved
- 1 tsp olive oil
- 1/4 tsp salt
- 1/4 tsp black pepper

Instructions:

1. Place the rice cakes on a plate or serving board.

2. In a small bowl, mash the avocado with a fork until smooth.

3. Spread the mashed avocado evenly over the rice cakes.

4. Arrange the halved cherry tomatoes on top of the avocado.

5. Drizzle the olive oil over the tomatoes.

6. Season with salt and black pepper.

That's it! This makes a simple, healthy, and delicious snack or light meal.

The creamy avocado pairs perfectly with the juicy cherry tomatoes, and the whole grain rice cakes provide a satisfying crunch. The olive oil, salt, and pepper add flavor and balance.

You can use any variety of rice cakes you prefer - plain, multigrain, or even flavored. Adjust the amount of avocado and tomatoes to your liking.

For extra flavor, you can also try:
- Sprinkling a bit of garlic powder or dried herbs over the top
- Squeezing a bit of lemon juice over the avocado
- Adding a sprinkle of feta or goat cheese

This is a quick, easy, and nutritious snack that's perfect for a light lunch or afternoon pick-me-up. Enjoy the combination of healthy fats, complex carbs, and fresh produce!

45. Chicken and vegetable soup

Ingredients:
- 1 lb boneless, skinless chicken breasts, cubed
- 1 tbsp olive oil
- 1 onion, diced
- 3 carrots, peeled and sliced
- 2 celery stalks, sliced
- 3 garlic cloves, minced
- 6 cups low-sodium chicken broth
- 1 (15 oz) can diced tomatoes
- 1 cup frozen green beans
- 1 cup frozen peas
- 1 tsp dried thyme
- 1 tsp dried oregano
- Salt and black pepper to taste

Instructions:

1. In a large pot or Dutch oven, heat the olive oil over medium heat. Add the chicken and cook for 3-4 minutes until lightly browned.

2. Add the onion, carrots, celery, and garlic. Sauté for 5 minutes until the vegetables start to soften.

3. Pour in the chicken broth and diced tomatoes. Bring to a boil.

4. Reduce heat to medium-low and stir in the green beans, peas, thyme, and oregano. Season with salt and pepper to taste.

5. Simmer the soup for 15-20 minutes, until the chicken is cooked through and the vegetables are tender.

6. Serve hot, garnished with extra herbs if desired.

This hearty chicken and vegetable soup is packed with protein, fiber, vitamins, and minerals. The combination of chicken, vegetables, and herbs creates a flavorful and nourishing meal.

You can use any mix of vegetables you prefer, such as zucchini, spinach, or corn. Adjust the seasoning to your taste.

This soup can be made ahead of time and reheated for easy lunches or dinners throughout the week. Enjoy!

46. Minestrone soup

Ingredients:
- 2 tbsp olive oil
- 1 onion, diced
- 3 carrots, peeled and diced
- 3 celery stalks, diced
- 4 garlic cloves, minced
- 1 tsp dried oregano
- 1 tsp dried basil
- 1/4 tsp red pepper flakes (optional)
- 1 (28 oz) can diced tomatoes
- 4 cups low-sodium vegetable or chicken broth
- 1 (15 oz) can kidney beans, drained and rinsed
- 1 (15 oz) can cannellini beans, drained and rinsed
- 2 cups chopped kale or spinach
- 1 cup small pasta (such as ditalini or elbow macaroni)
- Salt and black pepper to taste
- Grated Parmesan cheese for serving (optional)

Instructions:

1. In a large pot or Dutch oven, heat the olive oil over medium heat. Add the onion, carrots, celery, and garlic. Sauté for 5-7 minutes until the vegetables start to soften.

2. Stir in the oregano, basil, and red pepper flakes (if using). Cook for 1 minute until fragrant.

3. Pour in the diced tomatoes and broth. Bring the soup to a boil.

4. Reduce heat to medium-low and stir in the kidney beans, cannellini beans, kale/spinach, and pasta.

5. Simmer the soup for 15-20 minutes, until the pasta is tender. Season with salt and pepper to taste. Serve the minestrone soup hot, garnished with grated Parmesan cheese if desired.

This hearty, veggie-packed minestrone soup is a nutritious and comforting meal. The combination of beans, greens, and small pasta makes it satisfying and filling.

You can customize the vegetables and beans to your liking. Other great additions include zucchini, green beans, or pesto.

This soup can be made in advance and reheated for easy lunches or dinners throughout the week. Enjoy!

47. Butternut squash soup

Ingredients:
- 1 medium butternut squash, peeled, seeded, and cubed (about 4 cups)
- 1 tbsp olive oil
- 1 onion, diced
- 3 garlic cloves, minced
- 4 cups low-sodium vegetable or chicken broth
- 1 cup unsweetened almond milk (or regular milk)
- 1 tsp ground cumin
- 1/2 tsp ground cinnamon
- 1/4 tsp ground nutmeg
- Salt and black pepper to taste
- Chopped fresh parsley for garnish (optional)

Instructions:

1. In a large pot or Dutch oven, heat the olive oil over medium heat. Add the diced onion and sauté for 5 minutes until translucent.

2. Add the minced garlic and sauté for 1 minute until fragrant.

3. Add the cubed butternut squash and broth. Bring the mixture to a boil.

4. Reduce heat to medium-low and simmer for 20-25 minutes, until the squash is very soft.

5. Using an immersion blender, carefully blend the soup until smooth and creamy. Alternatively, you can transfer the soup in batches to a regular blender.

6. Stir in the almond milk, cumin, cinnamon, and nutmeg. Season with salt and pepper to taste.

7. Reheat the soup if needed and serve warm, garnished with chopped fresh parsley if desired.

This butternut squash soup is rich, creamy, and full of cozy fall flavors. The blend of spices complements the natural sweetness of the squash.

You can use regular dairy milk instead of almond milk if preferred. For a thicker consistency, use less broth or milk.

This soup can be made in advance and reheated. It also freezes well for easy meal prep. Enjoy this nourishing and delicious butternut squash soup!

48. Lentil and sweet potato stew

Ingredients:
- 1 tbsp olive oil
- 1 onion, diced
- 3 garlic cloves, minced
- 2 medium sweet potatoes, peeled and cubed
- 1 cup dried brown or green lentils, rinsed
- 4 cups low-sodium vegetable or chicken broth
- 1 (15 oz) can diced tomatoes
- 1 tsp ground cumin
- 1 tsp smoked paprika
- 1/2 tsp dried thyme
- Salt and black pepper to taste
- Chopped fresh parsley for garnish (optional)

Instructions:
1. In a large pot or Dutch oven, heat the olive oil over medium heat. Add the diced onion and sauté for 5 minutes until translucent.

2. Add the minced garlic and sauté for 1 minute until fragrant.

3. Stir in the cubed sweet potatoes, rinsed lentils, vegetable broth, and diced tomatoes.

4. Season with the cumin, smoked paprika, thyme, salt, and pepper. Stir to combine.

5. Bring the stew to a boil, then reduce heat to medium-low. Simmer for 25-30 minutes, stirring occasionally, until the lentils and sweet potatoes are tender.

6. Taste and adjust seasoning as needed. Serve the lentil and sweet potato stew hot, garnished with chopped fresh parsley if desired.

This hearty, nourishing stew is packed with plant-based protein from the lentils and complex carbs from the sweet potatoes. The blend of spices adds wonderful flavor.

You can use any type of lentils you prefer - brown, green, or red will all work well. Adjust the cooking time as needed based on the type of lentils used.

For extra creaminess, you can stir in a splash of unsweetened almond milk or coconut milk at the end.

This stew makes a satisfying and comforting meal on its own, or you can serve it with crusty bread or a fresh salad. Enjoy this delicious lentil and sweet potato stew!

49. Tomato and basil soup

Ingredients:
- 2 tbsp olive oil
- 1 onion, diced
- 3 garlic cloves, minced
- 2 (28 oz) cans diced tomatoes
- 2 cups low-sodium vegetable
or chicken broth
- 1/4 cup fresh basil leaves, chopped
- 1 tsp dried oregano
- 1/4 tsp red pepper flakes (optional)
- Salt and black pepper to taste
- Grated Parmesan cheese for serving (optional)

Instructions:

1. In a large pot or Dutch oven, heat the olive oil over medium heat. Add the diced onion and sauté for 5-7 minutes until translucent.

2. Add the minced garlic and sauté for 1 minute until fragrant.

3. Pour in the canned diced tomatoes and broth. Bring the mixture to a simmer.

4. Stir in the chopped fresh basil, dried oregano, and red pepper flakes (if using). Season with salt and pepper to taste.

5. Reduce heat to medium-low and let the soup simmer for 15-20 minutes, allowing the flavors to meld.

6. Using an immersion blender, carefully blend the soup until it reaches your desired consistency. Alternatively, you can transfer the soup in batches to a regular blender.

7. Taste and adjust seasoning as needed. Serve the tomato and basil soup hot, garnished with grated Parmesan cheese if desired.

This vibrant, flavorful soup captures the essence of fresh tomatoes and fragrant basil. The blend of aromatics, herbs, and spices creates a comforting and satisfying dish. For a creamier texture, you can stir in a splash of heavy cream or unsweetened almond milk at the end.

This soup can be made in advance and reheated for easy meals throughout the week. It also freezes well for longer-term storage.

Enjoy this delicious tomato and basil soup as a comforting lunch or dinner, paired with a fresh salad or crusty bread.

50. Beef and barley soup

Ingredients:
- 1 lb lean beef stew meat, cubed
- 2 tbsp olive oil
- 1 onion, diced
- 3 carrots, peeled and sliced
- 3 celery stalks, sliced
- 4 garlic cloves, minced
- 6 cups low-sodium beef or chicken broth
- 1 cup pearl barley, rinsed
- 1 (15 oz) can diced tomatoes
- 2 tsp dried thyme
- 1 tsp dried rosemary
- Salt and black pepper to taste
- Chopped fresh parsley for garnish (optional)

Instructions:
1. In a large pot or Dutch oven, heat the olive oil over medium-high heat. Add the cubed beef and brown on all sides, about 5 minutes total. Transfer the beef to a plate.

2. Reduce heat to medium and add the diced onion, sliced carrots, and celery to the pot. Sauté for 5-7 minutes until the vegetables start to soften.

3. Add the minced garlic and sauté for 1 minute until fragrant.

4. Pour in the beef broth and stir in the rinsed pearl barley. Bring the mixture to a boil.

5. Reduce heat to medium-low and add the browned beef, diced tomatoes, thyme, and rosemary. Season with salt and pepper.

6. Simmer the soup for 45-60 minutes, stirring occasionally, until the barley is tender and the beef is very soft.

7. Taste and adjust seasoning as needed. Serve the beef and barley soup hot, garnished with chopped fresh parsley if desired.

This hearty, nourishing soup is packed with tender beef, chewy barley, and an array of vegetables. The blend of herbs and spices creates a comforting, flavorful dish.

You can use any type of beef stew meat or chuck roast for this recipe. The long simmering time helps tenderize the meat.

For a thicker consistency, you can mash some of the cooked barley against the side of the pot. You can also add extra broth or water if the soup becomes too thick.

This soup makes a satisfying meal on its own, or you can serve it with crusty bread or a fresh salad. Enjoy this delicious beef and barley soup!

51. Spinach and white bean soup

Ingredients:
- 2 tbsp olive oil
- 1 onion, diced
- 3 garlic cloves, minced
- 2 carrots, peeled and sliced
- 2 celery stalks, sliced
- 4 cups low-sodium vegetable or chicken broth
- 1 (15 oz) can white beans, drained and rinsed
- 4 cups fresh spinach, chopped
- 1 tsp dried thyme
- 1/2 tsp dried rosemary
- Salt and black pepper to taste
- Grated Parmesan cheese for serving (optional)

Instructions:

1. In a large pot or Dutch oven, heat the olive oil over medium heat. Add the diced onion and sauté for 5 minutes until translucent.

2. Add the minced garlic, sliced carrots, and sliced celery. Sauté for 3-4 minutes until the vegetables start to soften.

3. Pour in the vegetable or chicken broth and bring the mixture to a simmer.

4. Stir in the drained and rinsed white beans, chopped spinach, dried thyme, and dried rosemary.

5. Season with salt and black pepper to taste.

6. Reduce heat to medium-low and let the soup simmer for 15-20 minutes, until the vegetables are tender and the flavors have melded.

7. Serve the spinach and white bean soup hot, garnished with grated Parmesan cheese if desired.

This nourishing soup is packed with protein-rich white beans, nutrient-dense spinach, and a variety of aromatic vegetables. The blend of herbs adds wonderful flavor.

You can use any type of white beans, such as cannellini, navy, or Great Northern beans. Adjust the amount of spinach to your preference.

For extra creaminess, you can stir in a splash of unsweetened almond milk or heavy cream at the end.

This soup makes a satisfying and comforting meal on its own, or you can serve it with crusty bread or a fresh salad. Enjoy this delicious spinach and white bean soup!

52. Carrot and ginger soup

Ingredients:
- 2 tbsp olive oil
- 1 onion, diced
- 3 garlic cloves, minced
- 1 lb carrots, peeled and sliced
- 4 cups low-sodium vegetable or chicken broth
- 1 cup unsweetened almond milk (or regular milk)
- 1 tsp ground cumin
- 1/2 tsp ground coriander
- Salt and black pepper to taste
- Chopped fresh parsley for garnish (optional)
- 1 tbsp grated fresh ginger

Instructions:

1. In a large pot or Dutch oven, heat the olive oil over medium heat. Add the diced onion and sauté for 5-7 minutes until translucent.

2. Add the minced garlic and grated ginger. Sauté for 1 minute until fragrant.

3. Stir in the sliced carrots and pour in the vegetable or chicken broth. Bring the mixture to a boil.

4. Reduce heat to medium-low and let the soup simmer for 20-25 minutes, until the carrots are very soft.

5. Using an immersion blender, carefully blend the soup until smooth and creamy. Alternatively, you can transfer the soup in batches to a regular blender.

6. Stir in the unsweetened almond milk, ground cumin, and ground coriander. Season with salt and black pepper to taste.

7. Reheat the soup if needed and serve warm, garnished with chopped fresh parsley if desired.

This vibrant, flavorful carrot and ginger soup is both nourishing and comforting. The ginger adds a nice kick of warmth and spice, while the carrots provide natural sweetness.

You can use regular dairy milk instead of almond milk if preferred. For a thicker consistency, use less milk or broth.

This soup can be made in advance and reheated for easy meals throughout the week. It also freezes well for longer-term storage.

Enjoy this creamy, delicious carrot and ginger soup as a healthy lunch or dinner, paired with crusty bread or a fresh salad.

53. Split pea soup with ham

Ingredients:
- 1 tbsp olive oil
- 1 onion, diced
- 3 carrots, peeled and diced
- 3 celery stalks, diced
- 3 garlic cloves, minced
- 1 lb dried split peas, rinsed
- 6 cups low-sodium chicken or vegetable broth
- 1 cup diced cooked ham
- 1 bay leaf
- 1 tsp dried thyme
- Salt and black pepper to taste

Instructions:

1. In a large pot or Dutch oven, heat the olive oil over medium heat. Add the diced onion, carrots, and celery. Sauté for 5-7 minutes until the vegetables start to soften.

2. Add the minced garlic and sauté for 1 minute until fragrant.

3. Stir in the rinsed split peas, chicken or vegetable broth, diced ham, bay leaf, and dried thyme.

4. Bring the soup to a boil, then reduce heat to medium-low. Simmer for 45-60 minutes, stirring occasionally, until the split peas are very soft and the soup has thickened.

5. Remove the bay leaf. Use an immersion blender to partially blend the soup, leaving some texture. Alternatively, you can transfer a portion of the soup to a regular blender and blend until smooth, then return it to the pot.

6. Season the split pea soup with salt and black pepper to taste. Serve the soup hot, garnished with extra diced ham or chopped parsley if desired.

This hearty split pea soup is packed with protein from the split peas and ham. The blend of aromatic vegetables and herbs creates a comforting, flavorful dish.

You can use any type of cooked ham, such as smoked, honey-baked, or diced ham steak. Adjust the amount to your preference. For a vegetarian version, simply omit the ham and use vegetable broth instead of chicken broth.

This soup makes a satisfying meal on its own, or you can serve it with crusty bread or a fresh salad. Enjoy this delicious split pea and ham soup!

54. Mushroom and wild rice soup

Ingredients:
- 1 cup wild rice, rinsed
- 8 cups vegetable or chicken broth
- 2 tablespoons olive oil
- 1 onion, finely chopped
- 3 cloves garlic, minced
- 1 lb (450g) mushrooms (such as cremini or button), sliced
- 2 carrots, diced
- 2 celery stalks, diced
- 1 teaspoon dried thyme
- 1 teaspoon dried rosemary
- Salt and pepper to taste
- 1/2 cup heavy cream (optional)
- Chopped fresh parsley for garnish (optional)

Instructions:
1. In a large pot, combine the wild rice and broth. Bring to a boil over medium-high heat. Reduce heat to low, cover, and simmer for 45 minutes to 1 hour, or until rice is tender.

2. In a separate large pot, heat the olive oil over medium heat. Add the onion and garlic, and sauté until softened and fragrant, about 3-4 minutes.

3. Add the sliced mushrooms to the pot and cook until they release their liquid and begin to brown, about 5-7 minutes.

4. Stir in the diced carrots, celery, thyme, and rosemary. Cook for an additional 5 minutes, until vegetables are slightly softened.

5. Once the wild rice is cooked, add it along with the broth to the pot with the vegetables. Stir to combine. If the soup seems too thick, you can add more broth or water to reach your desired consistency.

6. Season with salt and pepper to taste. If using heavy cream, stir it in at this point for added richness. Allow the soup to simmer for an additional 10-15 minutes to allow the flavors to meld together.

7. Serve hot, garnished with chopped fresh parsley if desired. Enjoy!

This soup is hearty and comforting, perfect for a cozy night in or as a starter for a special meal. Feel free to customize it with your favorite herbs or additional vegetables!

55. Cauliflower and leek soup

Ingredients:
- 1 large head of cauliflower, chopped into florets
- 2 leeks, white and light green parts only, chopped
- 2 cloves garlic, minced
- 1 onion, chopped
- 4 cups vegetable or chicken broth
- 1 cup milk or heavy cream
- 2 tablespoons olive oil
- 1 teaspoon dried thyme
- Salt and pepper to taste
- Chopped fresh chives or parsley for garnish (optional)

Instructions:
1. In a large pot, heat the olive oil over medium heat. Add the chopped onion and leeks. Sauté until softened, about 5 minutes.

2. Add the minced garlic to the pot and cook for an additional minute until fragrant.

3. Add the cauliflower florets to the pot along with the vegetable or chicken broth. Bring to a simmer and cook until the cauliflower is tender, about 15-20 minutes.

4. Once the cauliflower is tender, use an immersion blender or transfer the soup in batches to a blender to puree until smooth. Be careful when blending hot liquids.

5. Return the pureed soup to the pot if necessary. Stir in the milk or heavy cream, dried thyme, and season with salt and pepper to taste. Allow the soup to simmer for an additional 5-10 minutes to heat through and allow the flavors to meld together.

6. If the soup is too thick, you can thin it out with additional broth or water to reach your desired consistency.

7. Serve hot, garnished with chopped fresh chives or parsley if desired. Enjoy!

This creamy Cauliflower and Leek Soup is a comforting and nutritious dish that's perfect for any occasion. It's also easy to customize with your favorite herbs or spices to suit your taste preferences.

56. Kale and quinoa salad with cranberries

Ingredients:
- 1 cup quinoa
- 2 cups water or vegetable broth
- 4 cups kale, stems removed and chopped
- 1/2 cup dried cranberries
- 1/4 cup sliced almonds
- 1/4 cup crumbled feta cheese (optional)
- 2 tablespoons olive oil
- 2 tablespoons balsamic vinegar
- 1 tablespoon honey or maple syrup
- Salt and pepper to taste

Instructions:

1. Rinse the quinoa under cold water using a fine-mesh sieve. In a medium saucepan, combine the quinoa and water or vegetable broth. Bring to a boil, then reduce the heat to low, cover, and simmer for 15-20 minutes, or until the quinoa is cooked and fluffy. Remove from heat and let it cool slightly.

2. In a large mixing bowl, combine the chopped kale, cooked quinoa, dried cranberries, sliced almonds, and crumbled feta cheese (if using).

3. In a small bowl, whisk together the olive oil, balsamic vinegar, honey or maple syrup, salt, and pepper to make the dressing.

4. Pour the dressing over the kale and quinoa mixture, and toss until everything is evenly coated.

5. Allow the salad to sit for at least 10-15 minutes before serving to allow the flavors to meld together and the kale to soften slightly.

6. Serve the salad chilled or at room temperature. Enjoy!

This Kale and Quinoa Salad with Cranberries is packed with flavor and nutrients, making it a perfect option for a light lunch or a side dish for dinner. Feel free to customize it with your favorite toppings or add-ins, such as grilled chicken or avocado, to make it even more satisfying!

57. Cucumber and tomato salad with feta

Ingredients:
- 2 large cucumbers, diced
- 2 large tomatoes, diced
- 1/2 red onion, thinly sliced
- 1/4 cup crumbled feta cheese
- 2 tablespoons fresh lemon juice
- 2 tablespoons extra virgin olive oil
- 1 tablespoon chopped fresh parsley
- 1 tablespoon chopped fresh dill (optional)
- Salt and pepper to taste

Instructions:

1. In a large mixing bowl, combine the diced cucumbers, diced tomatoes, and thinly sliced red onion.

2. In a small bowl, whisk together the fresh lemon juice, extra virgin olive oil, chopped parsley, chopped dill (if using), salt, and pepper to make the dressing.

3. Pour the dressing over the cucumber, tomato, and onion mixture, and toss gently to coat everything evenly.

4. Add the crumbled feta cheese to the salad and toss lightly to distribute it throughout.

5. Taste and adjust the seasoning with additional salt, pepper, or lemon juice if needed.

6. Serve the salad immediately, or chill it in the refrigerator for at least 30 minutes to allow the flavors to meld together before serving.

7. Enjoy this refreshing and flavorful Cucumber and Tomato Salad with Feta as a side dish or a light meal on its own!

This salad is perfect for summer gatherings, barbecues, or as a quick and healthy side dish for any meal. The combination of crisp cucumbers, juicy tomatoes, tangy feta cheese, and zesty dressing is sure to be a hit!

58. Beet and arugula salad with walnuts

Ingredients:
- 3 medium beets, cooked, peeled, and thinly sliced
- 4 cups fresh arugula
- 1/2 cup walnuts, toasted and chopped
- 1/4 cup crumbled goat cheese or feta cheese (optional)
- 2 tablespoons balsamic vinegar
- 2 tablespoons extra virgin olive oil
- 1 tablespoon honey or maple syrup
- Salt and pepper to taste

Instructions:

1. Start by preparing the beets. You can cook them by boiling, roasting, or steaming until tender. Once cooked, let them cool slightly, then peel and thinly slice them.

2. In a large mixing bowl, combine the sliced beets, fresh arugula, and toasted chopped walnuts.

3. In a small bowl, whisk together the balsamic vinegar, extra virgin olive oil, honey or maple syrup, salt, and pepper to make the dressing.

4. Drizzle the dressing over the beet and arugula mixture, and toss gently to coat everything evenly.

5. If using, sprinkle the crumbled goat cheese or feta cheese over the salad and toss lightly to distribute.

6. Taste and adjust the seasoning with additional salt, pepper, or vinegar if needed.

7. Serve the salad immediately, garnished with additional walnuts or cheese if desired.

8. Enjoy this vibrant and flavorful Beet and Arugula Salad with Walnuts as a light lunch or a side dish for dinner!

This salad combines the earthy sweetness of beets with the peppery bite of arugula and the crunchy texture of toasted walnuts for a delicious and nutritious dish. It's perfect for any occasion and is sure to impress!

59. Roasted chickpea and avocado salad

Ingredients:
- 1 can (15 oz) chickpeas (garbanzo beans), drained and rinsed
- 2 ripe avocados, diced
- 1 cup cherry tomatoes, halved
- 1/4 red onion, thinly sliced
- 2 cups mixed greens (such as spinach, arugula, or lettuce)
- 2 tablespoons olive oil
- 1 teaspoon ground cumin
- 1 teaspoon paprika
- 1/2 teaspoon garlic powder
- Salt and pepper to taste
- Juice of 1 lemon or lime
- Optional toppings: crumbled feta cheese, chopped fresh cilantro, or toasted sesame seeds

Instructions:
1. Preheat your oven to 400°F (200°C).

2. In a bowl, toss the drained and rinsed chickpeas with olive oil, ground cumin, paprika, garlic powder, salt, and pepper until evenly coated.

3. Spread the seasoned chickpeas in a single layer on a baking sheet lined with parchment paper. Roast in the preheated oven for 20-25 minutes, or until the chickpeas are crispy and golden brown. Remove from the oven and let them cool slightly.

4. In a large salad bowl, combine the mixed greens, diced avocado, halved cherry tomatoes, and thinly sliced red onion.

5. Add the roasted chickpeas to the salad bowl.

6. Drizzle the salad with the juice of 1 lemon or lime, and toss gently to combine.

7. Taste and adjust the seasoning with additional salt, pepper, or lemon/lime juice if needed.

8. If desired, sprinkle the salad with crumbled feta cheese, chopped fresh cilantro, or toasted sesame seeds for added flavor and texture. Serve immediately and enjoy this delicious and nutritious Roasted Chickpea and Avocado Salad!

This salad is packed with protein, fiber, and healthy fats, making it a satisfying and flavorful meal or side dish. It's perfect for lunch or dinner and can be easily customized with your favorite toppings or dressings.

60. Spinach, strawberry, and walnut salad

Ingredients:
- 6 cups fresh baby spinach leaves
- 1 pint strawberries, hulled and sliced
- 1/2 cup walnuts, chopped and toasted
- 1/4 cup crumbled feta cheese (optional)
- 2 tablespoons balsamic vinegar
- 2 tablespoons extra virgin olive oil
- 1 tablespoon honey or maple syrup
- Salt and pepper to taste

Instructions:

1. In a large salad bowl, combine the fresh baby spinach leaves, sliced strawberries, and chopped toasted walnuts.

2. If using, sprinkle the crumbled feta cheese over the salad.

3. In a small bowl, whisk together the balsamic vinegar, extra virgin olive oil, honey or maple syrup, salt, and pepper to make the dressing.

4. Drizzle the dressing over the spinach, strawberry, and walnut mixture, and toss gently to coat everything evenly.

5. Taste and adjust the seasoning with additional salt, pepper, or vinegar if needed.

6. Serve the salad immediately as a refreshing and nutritious side dish or light meal.

7. Enjoy this vibrant and flavorful Spinach, Strawberry, and Walnut Salad!

This salad is perfect for spring and summer gatherings, picnics, or as a light and healthy meal any time of the year. The combination of sweet strawberries, crunchy walnuts, and tangy balsamic dressing is simply irresistible!

61. Arugula and pear salad with blue cheese

Ingredients:
- 4 cups fresh arugula
- 2 ripe pears, thinly sliced
- 1/2 cup crumbled blue cheese
- 1/4 cup chopped walnuts or pecans, toasted
- 2 tablespoons extra virgin olive oil
- 1 tablespoon balsamic vinegar
- 1 teaspoon honey or maple syrup
- Salt and pepper to taste

Instructions:
1. In a large salad bowl, combine the fresh arugula, thinly sliced pears, crumbled blue cheese, and toasted chopped walnuts or pecans.

2. In a small bowl, whisk together the extra virgin olive oil, balsamic vinegar, honey or maple syrup, salt, and pepper to make the dressing.

3. Drizzle the dressing over the arugula, pear, blue cheese, and walnut mixture, and toss gently to coat everything evenly.

4. Taste and adjust the seasoning with additional salt, pepper, or vinegar if needed.

5. Serve the salad immediately as a refreshing and flavorful side dish or light meal.

6. Enjoy this elegant and satisfying Arugula and Pear Salad with Blue Cheese!

This salad is perfect for special occasions or everyday meals. The peppery arugula, sweet and juicy pears, creamy blue cheese, and crunchy nuts create a perfect balance of flavors and textures. It's sure to impress your family and friends!

62. Greek salad with olives and feta

Ingredients:
- 4 medium tomatoes, chopped
- 1 cucumber, chopped
- 1 red onion, thinly sliced
- 1/2 green bell pepper, chopped
- 1/2 cup Kalamata olives, pitted
- 1/2 cup crumbled feta cheese
- 2 tablespoons extra virgin olive oil
- 1 tablespoon red wine vinegar
- 1 teaspoon dried oregano
- Salt and pepper to taste

Instructions:
1. In a large salad bowl, combine the chopped tomatoes, cucumber, red onion, and green bell pepper.

2. Add the pitted Kalamata olives to the bowl.

3. In a small bowl, whisk together the extra virgin olive oil, red wine vinegar, dried oregano, salt, and pepper to make the dressing.

4. Drizzle the dressing over the salad ingredients in the bowl, and toss gently to coat everything evenly.

5. Sprinkle the crumbled feta cheese over the top of the salad.

6. Taste and adjust the seasoning with additional salt, pepper, or vinegar if needed.

7. Serve the Greek Salad immediately as a refreshing and flavorful side dish or light meal.

8. Enjoy this classic and delicious Greek Salad with Olives and Feta!

This salad is bursting with Mediterranean flavors and is perfect for any occasion. It's simple to make yet incredibly satisfying, making it a favorite among many. Serve it alongside grilled meats, fish, or enjoy it on its own as a light and healthy meal.

63. Roasted vegetable and farro salad

Ingredients:
- 1 cup farro
- 2 cups water or vegetable broth
- 2 cups mixed vegetables (such as bell peppers, zucchini, cherry tomatoes, red onion, and carrots), chopped
- 2 tablespoons olive oil
- Salt and pepper to taste
- 1/4 cup chopped fresh herbs (such as parsley, basil, or thyme)
- 1/4 cup crumbled feta cheese or goat cheese (optional)
- Balsamic glaze for drizzling (optional)

Instructions:
1. Preheat your oven to 400°F (200°C).

2. Rinse the farro under cold water using a fine-mesh sieve. In a medium saucepan, combine the farro and water or vegetable broth. Bring to a boil, then reduce the heat to low, cover, and simmer for 25-30 minutes, or until the farro is tender and all the liquid is absorbed. Remove from heat and let it cool slightly.

3. While the farro is cooking, spread the chopped mixed vegetables on a baking sheet lined with parchment paper. Drizzle with olive oil and season with salt and pepper to taste. Toss to coat the vegetables evenly.

4. Roast the vegetables in the preheated oven for 20-25 minutes, or until they are tender and slightly caramelized, stirring halfway through.

5. In a large mixing bowl, combine the cooked farro and roasted vegetables. Add the chopped fresh herbs and toss gently to combine.

6. If using, sprinkle the crumbled feta cheese or goat cheese over the salad.

7. Drizzle with balsamic glaze, if desired, for added flavor. Taste and adjust the seasoning with additional salt and pepper if needed.

8. Serve the Roasted Vegetable and Farro Salad warm or at room temperature as a delicious and satisfying meal. Enjoy this hearty and nutritious salad as a main course or side dish!

This Roasted Vegetable and Farro Salad is packed with fiber, vitamins, and minerals, making it a nutritious and filling option for lunch or dinner. It's also versatile, so feel free to customize it with your favorite vegetables and toppings.

64. Caesar salad with grilled chicken

Ingredients:
For the Dressing:
- 1/2 cup mayonnaise
- 2 cloves garlic, minced
- 2 anchovy fillets, minced
(optional, but traditional)
- 1 tablespoon Dijon mustard
- 2 tablespoons freshly squeezed lemon juice
- 1/4 cup grated Parmesan cheese
- 1/4 cup extra virgin olive oil
- Salt and pepper to taste

For the Salad:
- 2 boneless, skinless chicken breasts
- Salt and pepper to taste
- 1 tablespoon olive oil
- 1 large head of romaine lettuce,
washed and chopped
- 1/2 cup croutons
- 1/4 cup grated Parmesan cheese
- Optional: additional Parmesan
cheese shavings for garnish

Instructions:
1. Preheat your grill or grill pan to medium-high heat.

2. Season the chicken breasts with salt, pepper, and olive oil. Grill the chicken for about 6-8 minutes per side, or until cooked through and no longer pink in the center. Remove from the grill and let them rest for a few minutes before slicing.

3. While the chicken is grilling, prepare the dressing. In a small bowl, whisk together the mayonnaise, minced garlic, minced anchovy fillets (if using), Dijon mustard, lemon juice, grated Parmesan cheese, and extra virgin olive oil until well combined. Season with salt and pepper to taste.

4. In a large salad bowl, toss the chopped romaine lettuce with the croutons and grated Parmesan cheese.

5. Add the sliced grilled chicken to the salad bowl.

6. Drizzle the Caesar dressing over the salad, and toss gently to coat everything evenly.

7. Taste and adjust the seasoning with additional salt, pepper, or lemon juice if needed.

8. If desired, garnish the salad with additional Parmesan cheese shavings. Serve the Caesar Salad with Grilled Chicken immediately as a delicious and satisfying main course. Enjoy this classic and flavorful salad!

This Caesar Salad with Grilled Chicken is perfect for a light and satisfying meal. The combination of crisp romaine lettuce, juicy grilled chicken, crunchy croutons, and creamy Caesar dressing is simply irresistible!

65. Caprese salad with fresh basil

Ingredients:
- 4 large ripe tomatoes, sliced
- 1 pound fresh mozzarella cheese, sliced
- 1/4 cup fresh basil leaves
- Extra virgin olive oil, for drizzling
- Balsamic glaze, for drizzling (optional)
- Salt and pepper to taste

Instructions:

1. Arrange the sliced tomatoes and fresh mozzarella cheese on a serving platter, alternating them in a single layer.

2. Tuck fresh basil leaves in between the tomato and mozzarella slices.

3. Drizzle extra virgin olive oil over the tomatoes, mozzarella, and basil leaves.

4. If desired, drizzle balsamic glaze over the salad for added flavor.

5. Season the salad with salt and pepper to taste.

6. Serve the Caprese Salad with Fresh Basil immediately as a refreshing and elegant appetizer or side dish.

7. Enjoy this classic Italian salad with its vibrant colors and flavors!

This Caprese Salad with Fresh Basil is perfect for showcasing the delicious flavors of ripe tomatoes, creamy mozzarella cheese, and aromatic basil. It's a light and refreshing dish that's perfect for summer gatherings, picnics, or anytime you want a taste of Italy!

66. Mixed greens with roasted beets and goat cheese

Ingredients:
- 4 medium beets, washed, peeled, and cubed
- 6 cups mixed salad greens (such as spinach, arugula, and mesclun)
- 1/2 cup crumbled goat cheese
- 1/4 cup chopped walnuts or pecans, toasted
- 2 tablespoons extra virgin olive oil
- 1 tablespoon balsamic vinegar
- 1 teaspoon honey or maple syrup
- Salt and pepper to taste

Instructions:
1. Preheat your oven to 400°F (200°C).

2. Place the cubed beets on a baking sheet lined with parchment paper. Drizzle with olive oil and season with salt and pepper to taste. Toss to coat the beets evenly.

3. Roast the beets in the preheated oven for 25-30 minutes, or until they are tender and caramelized, stirring halfway through. Remove from the oven and let them cool slightly.

4. In a large salad bowl, combine the mixed salad greens, roasted beets, crumbled goat cheese, and toasted chopped walnuts or pecans.

5. In a small bowl, whisk together the extra virgin olive oil, balsamic vinegar, honey or maple syrup, salt, and pepper to make the dressing.

6. Drizzle the dressing over the salad ingredients in the bowl, and toss gently to coat everything evenly.

7. Taste and adjust the seasoning with additional salt, pepper, or vinegar if needed.

8. Serve the Mixed Greens Salad with Roasted Beets and Goat Cheese immediately as a delicious and nutritious side dish or light meal.

9. Enjoy this flavorful and colorful salad!

This Mixed Greens Salad with Roasted Beets and Goat Cheese is both elegant and delicious. The combination of sweet and earthy roasted beets, creamy goat cheese, and crunchy nuts pairs perfectly with the fresh mixed greens and tangy balsamic dressing. It's sure to be a hit at any meal!

67. Steamed broccoli with lemon

Ingredients:
- 1 large head of broccoli, cut into florets
- 2 tablespoons butter or olive oil
- Zest of 1 lemon
- Juice of 1 lemon
- Salt and pepper to taste

Instructions:
1. Fill a large pot with about 1 inch of water and place a steamer basket inside. Bring the water to a boil over medium-high heat.

2. Add the broccoli florets to the steamer basket, cover the pot, and steam for about 5-7 minutes, or until the broccoli is tender but still bright green.

3. While the broccoli is steaming, melt the butter in a small saucepan over medium heat. Once melted, remove from heat and stir in the lemon zest and lemon juice.

4. Once the broccoli is cooked, transfer it to a serving dish. Pour the lemon butter mixture over the broccoli and toss gently to coat.

5. Season the broccoli with salt and pepper to taste.

6. Serve the Steamed Broccoli with Lemon immediately as a flavorful and nutritious side dish.

7. Enjoy the bright and zesty flavors of this simple and healthy dish!

This Steamed Broccoli with Lemon is a quick and easy way to elevate plain steamed broccoli into a flavorful side dish. The combination of tender broccoli with the tangy freshness of lemon is sure to brighten up any meal.

68. Roasted sweet potato wedges

Ingredients:
- 2 large sweet potatoes, scrubbed and cut into wedges
- 2 tablespoons olive oil
- 1 teaspoon paprika
- 1/2 teaspoon garlic powder
- 1/2 teaspoon onion powder
- Salt and pepper to taste
- Optional: chopped fresh herbs such as rosemary or thyme for garnish

Instructions:
1. Preheat your oven to 425°F (220°C).

2. In a large bowl, toss the sweet potato wedges with olive oil, paprika, garlic powder, onion powder, salt, and pepper until evenly coated.

3. Arrange the seasoned sweet potato wedges in a single layer on a baking sheet lined with parchment paper.

4. Roast the sweet potato wedges in the preheated oven for 25-30 minutes, flipping halfway through, or until they are tender and golden brown.

5. Once roasted, remove the sweet potato wedges from the oven and transfer them to a serving dish.

6. Optional: Garnish the roasted sweet potato wedges with chopped fresh herbs such as rosemary or thyme for added flavor and freshness.

7. Serve the roasted sweet potato wedges hot as a delicious and nutritious side dish or snack.

8. Enjoy the crispy and flavorful roasted sweet potato wedges!

These roasted sweet potato wedges are naturally sweet, crispy on the outside, and tender on the inside. They're perfect for serving alongside your favorite main dishes or as a tasty snack on their own. Feel free to customize the seasoning to your taste preferences!

69. Quinoa pilaf with herbs

Ingredients:
- 1 cup quinoa, rinsed
- 2 cups vegetable or chicken broth
- 2 tablespoons olive oil
- 1 onion, finely chopped
- 2 cloves garlic, minced
- 1/2 cup chopped mixed herbs (such as parsley, cilantro, dill, and mint)
- Salt and pepper to taste
- Optional: lemon zest for garnish

Instructions:
1. In a fine-mesh sieve, rinse the quinoa under cold water until the water runs clear.

2. In a medium saucepan, combine the rinsed quinoa and broth. Bring to a boil over medium-high heat, then reduce the heat to low, cover, and simmer for about 15-20 minutes, or until the quinoa is cooked and the liquid is absorbed.

3. While the quinoa is cooking, heat the olive oil in a large skillet over medium heat. Add the chopped onion and cook until softened, about 5 minutes.

4. Add the minced garlic to the skillet and cook for an additional minute until fragrant.

5. Once the quinoa is cooked, fluff it with a fork and transfer it to the skillet with the onion and garlic.

6. Add the chopped mixed herbs to the skillet and toss everything together until well combined.

7. Season the quinoa pilaf with salt and pepper to taste.

8. Optional: Garnish the quinoa pilaf with lemon zest for a fresh burst of flavor.

9. Serve the quinoa pilaf hot as a flavorful and nutritious side dish.

10. Enjoy the aromatic and herb-infused quinoa pilaf!

This quinoa pilaf with herbs is packed with flavor and makes a great accompaniment to a variety of main dishes. It's also versatile, so feel free to customize it with your favorite herbs and spices.

70. Brown rice with black beans

Ingredients:
- 1 cup brown rice
- 2 cups water or vegetable broth
- 1 can (15 oz) black beans, drained and rinsed
- 1 tablespoon olive oil
- 1 small onion, diced
- 2 cloves garlic, minced
- 1 teaspoon ground cumin
- 1 teaspoon chili powder
- Salt and pepper to taste
- Optional toppings: chopped fresh cilantro, diced avocado, salsa, lime wedges

Instructions:
1. Rinse the brown rice under cold water using a fine-mesh sieve. In a medium saucepan, combine the brown rice and water or vegetable broth. Bring to a boil, then reduce the heat to low, cover, and simmer for about 45-50 minutes, or until the rice is cooked and the liquid is absorbed.

2. While the rice is cooking, heat the olive oil in a large skillet over medium heat. Add the diced onion and cook until softened, about 5 minutes.

3. Add the minced garlic to the skillet and cook for an additional minute until fragrant.

4. Stir in the drained and rinsed black beans, ground cumin, and chili powder. Cook for a few minutes until the beans are heated through and the spices are fragrant. Season with salt and pepper to taste.

5. Once the rice is cooked, fluff it with a fork and transfer it to the skillet with the black beans mixture. Stir everything together until well combined.

6. Taste and adjust the seasoning if needed. Serve the Brown Rice with Black Beans hot as a satisfying and nutritious main dish or side dish.

7. Optional: Garnish with chopped fresh cilantro, diced avocado, salsa, or a squeeze of lime juice for added flavor. Enjoy this hearty and flavorful Brown Rice with Black Beans!

This dish is not only tasty but also packed with protein, fiber, and essential nutrients. It's a versatile and budget-friendly meal that's perfect for busy weeknights or meal prep. Feel free to customize it with your favorite toppings or spices!

71. Grilled asparagus with balsamic glaze

Ingredients:
- 1 pound (about 450g) asparagus spears, woody ends trimmed
- 2 tablespoons olive oil
- Salt and pepper to taste
- Balsamic glaze for drizzling

Instructions:

1. Preheat your grill to medium-high heat.

2. In a large bowl, toss the trimmed asparagus spears with olive oil until evenly coated. Season with salt and pepper to taste.

3. Place the asparagus spears on the preheated grill in a single layer. Grill for about 3-5 minutes per side, or until the asparagus is tender and has grill marks.

4. Once the asparagus is grilled to your desired level of doneness, remove it from the grill and transfer it to a serving platter.

5. Drizzle the grilled asparagus with balsamic glaze.

6. Serve the Grilled Asparagus with Balsamic Glaze immediately as a delicious and flavorful side dish.

7. Enjoy the smoky flavor of the grilled asparagus paired with the sweet and tangy balsamic glaze!

This dish is not only tasty but also visually appealing, making it a great addition to any meal. It's quick and easy to prepare, and the balsamic glaze adds a touch of elegance to the dish. Serve it alongside grilled meats, fish, or as part of a vegetarian meal.

72. Roasted Brussels sprouts with garlic

Ingredients:
- 1 pound Brussels sprouts, trimmed and halved
- 3 tablespoons olive oil
- 4 cloves garlic, minced
- Salt and pepper to taste
- Optional: grated Parmesan cheese, lemon zest, or balsamic glaze for garnish

Instructions:
1. Preheat your oven to 400°F (200°C).

2. In a large bowl, toss the trimmed and halved Brussels sprouts with olive oil until evenly coated.

3. Add the minced garlic to the bowl and toss again to evenly distribute.

4. Spread the Brussels sprouts out in a single layer on a baking sheet lined with parchment paper.

5. Season the Brussels sprouts with salt and pepper to taste.

6. Roast the Brussels sprouts in the preheated oven for 20-25 minutes, stirring halfway through, or until they are tender and caramelized.

7. Once roasted, remove the Brussels sprouts from the oven and transfer them to a serving dish.

8. Optional: Garnish the roasted Brussels sprouts with grated Parmesan cheese, lemon zest, or a drizzle of balsamic glaze for added flavor and presentation.

9. Serve the Roasted Brussels Sprouts with Garlic hot as a delicious and nutritious side dish.

10. Enjoy the crispy and flavorful roasted Brussels sprouts!

These roasted Brussels sprouts with garlic make a wonderful addition to any meal. They're crispy on the outside, tender on the inside, and packed with savory garlic flavor. Serve them alongside roasted meats, grilled chicken, or as part of a vegetarian spread.

73. Cauliflower rice

Ingredients:
- 1 medium head of cauliflower
- 1 tablespoon olive oil or butter
- Salt and pepper to taste

Instructions:

1. Wash the cauliflower and pat it dry. Remove the leaves and cut the cauliflower into florets.

2. Working in batches, place the cauliflower florets in a food processor and pulse until they resemble rice-like grains. Be careful not to over-process, or you'll end up with cauliflower puree.

3. Heat the olive oil or butter in a large skillet over medium heat.

4. Add the riced cauliflower to the skillet and cook, stirring occasionally, for about 5-7 minutes, or until it's tender but still slightly crisp.

5. Season the cauliflower rice with salt and pepper to taste.

6. Once cooked, remove the cauliflower rice from the skillet and transfer it to a serving dish.

7. Serve the cauliflower rice hot as a delicious and nutritious side dish.

Cauliflower rice can be served as a base for stir-fries, curries, or as a substitute for rice in any recipe. You can also customize it by adding herbs, spices, or other flavorings to suit your taste preferences. Enjoy experimenting with this versatile and healthy ingredient!

74. Sautéed spinach with garlic

Ingredients:
- 1 tablespoon olive oil
- 2 cloves garlic, minced
- 8 cups fresh spinach leaves, washed and stems removed
- Salt and pepper to taste
- Optional: red pepper flakes for a bit of heat, lemon zest for brightness

Instructions:
1. Heat the olive oil in a large skillet over medium heat.

2. Add the minced garlic to the skillet and sauté for about 1 minute, or until fragrant.

3. Add the fresh spinach leaves to the skillet in batches, stirring continuously, until all the spinach is wilted. This should take about 2-3 minutes.

4. Season the sautéed spinach with salt and pepper to taste. If desired, add red pepper flakes for a bit of heat or lemon zest for brightness.

5. Once the spinach is wilted and tender, remove the skillet from the heat.

6. Transfer the sautéed spinach to a serving dish and serve immediately.

7. Enjoy this flavorful and nutritious side dish alongside your favorite main courses.

Sautéed spinach with garlic is a simple and healthy way to enjoy this nutritious leafy green. It's quick to make and packed with flavor, making it a great addition to any meal. Feel free to customize it with your favorite herbs or spices to suit your taste preferences!

75. Mashed sweet potatoes

Ingredients:
- 2 pounds sweet potatoes, peeled and cut into chunks
- 4 tablespoons unsalted butter, softened
- 1/4 cup milk (or dairy-free alternative)
- Salt and pepper to taste
- Optional toppings: chopped fresh herbs (such as parsley or chives), toasted pecans or walnuts, maple syrup, cinnamon

Instructions:
1. Place the sweet potato chunks in a large pot and cover them with cold water. Bring the water to a boil over medium-high heat, then reduce the heat to medium-low and simmer for about 15-20 minutes, or until the sweet potatoes are tender when pierced with a fork.

2. Drain the cooked sweet potatoes and return them to the pot.

3. Add the softened butter and milk to the pot with the sweet potatoes.

4. Use a potato masher or fork to mash the sweet potatoes until smooth and creamy. If you prefer a smoother texture, you can use a hand mixer or immersion blender.

5. Season the mashed sweet potatoes with salt and pepper to taste. Adjust the amount of butter and milk to achieve your desired consistency.

6. Transfer the mashed sweet potatoes to a serving dish.

7. Optional: Garnish the mashed sweet potatoes with chopped fresh herbs, toasted pecans or walnuts, a drizzle of maple syrup, or a sprinkle of cinnamon for added flavor and presentation.

8. Serve the mashed sweet potatoes hot as a delicious and nutritious side dish.

Mashed sweet potatoes are a cozy and comforting addition to any meal, especially during the fall and winter months. They're naturally sweet, creamy, and packed with vitamins and fiber. Enjoy them alongside roasted meats, poultry, or as part of a vegetarian spread.

76. Grilled zucchini and squash

Ingredients:
- 2 medium zucchinis, sliced lengthwise into 1/4-inch thick strips
- 2 medium yellow squash, sliced lengthwise into 1/4-inch thick strips
- 2 tablespoons olive oil
- 2 cloves garlic, minced
- Salt and pepper to taste
- Optional: chopped fresh herbs (such as basil or parsley), grated Parmesan cheese, balsamic glaze

Instructions:

1. Preheat your grill to medium-high heat.

2. In a small bowl, whisk together the olive oil and minced garlic.

3. Brush both sides of the zucchini and squash slices with the olive oil and garlic mixture. Season with salt and pepper to taste.

4. Place the zucchini and squash slices on the preheated grill in a single layer.

5. Grill the zucchini and squash for about 3-4 minutes per side, or until they are tender and have grill marks.

6. Once grilled, remove the zucchini and squash slices from the grill and transfer them to a serving platter.

7. Optional: Garnish the grilled zucchini and squash with chopped fresh herbs, grated Parmesan cheese, or a drizzle of balsamic glaze for added flavor and presentation.

8. Serve the grilled zucchini and squash hot as a delicious and nutritious side dish.

Grilled zucchini and squash are versatile and flavorful, making them a great addition to any meal. Enjoy them alongside grilled meats, poultry, or fish, or use them to top salads, sandwiches, or pizzas. They're quick and easy to make, and the grill adds a delicious smoky flavor to the vegetables.

77. Whole grain couscous with vegetables

Ingredients:
- 1 cup whole grain couscous
- 1 1/4 cups vegetable broth or water
- 2 tablespoons olive oil
- 1 small onion, diced
- 2 cloves garlic, minced
- 1 medium zucchini, diced
- 1 medium yellow squash, diced
- 1 bell pepper (any color), diced
- 1 cup cherry tomatoes, halved
- 1 teaspoon dried oregano
- 1 teaspoon dried thyme
- Salt and pepper to taste
- Optional: chopped fresh parsley or basil for garnish

Instructions:

1. In a medium saucepan, bring the vegetable broth or water to a boil.

2. Once boiling, stir in the whole grain couscous. Remove the saucepan from heat, cover, and let it sit for about 5 minutes, or until the couscous has absorbed all the liquid and is tender.

3. While the couscous is cooking, heat the olive oil in a large skillet over medium heat. Add the diced onion to the skillet and cook until softened, about 5 minutes. Add the minced garlic to the skillet and cook for an additional minute until fragrant.

4. Stir in the diced zucchini, yellow squash, and bell pepper. Cook for about 5-7 minutes, or until the vegetables are tender but still slightly crisp.

5. Add the halved cherry tomatoes to the skillet and cook for another 2-3 minutes, or until they are just starting to soften.

6. Sprinkle the dried oregano and thyme over the vegetables. Season with salt and pepper to taste.

7. Fluff the cooked couscous with a fork and transfer it to the skillet with the cooked vegetables. Toss everything together until well combined.

8. Optional: Garnish the whole grain couscous with chopped fresh parsley or basil for added flavor and freshness.

9. Serve the whole grain couscous with vegetables hot as a delicious and nutritious main dish or side dish.

Whole grain couscous with vegetables is a satisfying and versatile dish that's perfect for lunch or dinner. It's packed with fiber, vitamins, and minerals, making it a healthy choice for any meal. Enjoy it on its own or alongside grilled meats, poultry, or fish.

78. Greek yogurt with honey and nuts

Ingredients:
- 1 cup Greek yogurt
- 1-2 tablespoons honey (adjust to taste)
- 2 tablespoons chopped nuts (such as almonds, walnuts, or pecans)
- Optional: fresh fruit (such as berries or sliced bananas), granola, cinnamon

Instructions:
1. Spoon the Greek yogurt into a serving bowl or individual serving cups.

2. Drizzle the honey over the Greek yogurt, using as much or as little as you like depending on your preference for sweetness.

3. Sprinkle the chopped nuts over the Greek yogurt and honey.

4. Optional: Add fresh fruit, granola, or a sprinkle of cinnamon for extra flavor and texture.

5. Serve the Greek yogurt with honey and nuts immediately as a delicious and satisfying snack or dessert.

6. Enjoy the creamy texture of the Greek yogurt combined with the sweetness of the honey and the crunch of the nuts!

Greek yogurt with honey and nuts is not only delicious but also packed with protein, calcium, and healthy fats. It's a great way to satisfy your sweet tooth while still enjoying a nutritious treat. Feel free to customize it with your favorite toppings or add-ins to suit your taste preferences!

79. Baked apples with cinnamon

Ingredients:
- 4 large apples (such as Granny Smith or Honeycrisp), cored
- 2 tablespoons unsalted butter, melted
- 2 tablespoons brown sugar or maple syrup
- 1 teaspoon ground cinnamon
- Optional toppings: chopped nuts (such as walnuts or pecans), raisins, granola, vanilla ice cream

Instructions:

1. Preheat your oven to 375°F (190°C).

2. Use a paring knife or apple corer to remove the cores from the apples, leaving the bottoms intact. You can also use a melon baller or spoon to scoop out the cores.

3. Place the cored apples in a baking dish or on a baking sheet lined with parchment paper.

4. In a small bowl, mix together the melted butter, brown sugar or maple syrup, and ground cinnamon until well combined.

5. Spoon the butter mixture into the cavities of the cored apples, dividing it evenly among them.

6. Optional: Sprinkle chopped nuts, raisins, or granola over the top of each apple for added flavor and texture.

7. Bake the apples in the preheated oven for about 25-30 minutes, or until they are tender and the tops are slightly caramelized.

8. Once baked, remove the apples from the oven and let them cool slightly before serving.

9. Serve the baked apples with cinnamon hot as a delicious and comforting dessert.

10. Optional: Top each baked apple with a scoop of vanilla ice cream for an extra special treat.

Baked apples with cinnamon are a simple yet delightful dessert that's sure to please. They're naturally sweet and fragrant, with the warm spices of cinnamon adding a cozy touch. Enjoy them on their own or with your favorite toppings for a delicious treat!

80. Chia seed pudding with berries

Ingredients:
- 1/4 cup chia seeds
- 1 cup unsweetened almond milk (or any milk of your choice)
- 1 tablespoon maple syrup or honey (optional, for sweetness)
- 1/2 teaspoon vanilla extract
- 1 cup mixed berries (such as strawberries, blueberries, raspberries)

Instructions:
1. In a mixing bowl or jar, combine the chia seeds, unsweetened almond milk, maple syrup or honey (if using), and vanilla extract. Stir well to combine.

2. Let the chia seed mixture sit for about 5 minutes, then stir again to break up any clumps. This will prevent the chia seeds from clumping together as they absorb the liquid.

3. Cover the bowl or jar and refrigerate the chia seed mixture for at least 2 hours, or preferably overnight. This will allow the chia seeds to absorb the liquid and thicken into a pudding-like consistency.

4. Once the chia seed pudding has set, give it a good stir to break up any clumps.

5. Divide the chia seed pudding into serving bowls or glasses.

6. Top the chia seed pudding with mixed berries, arranging them as desired.

7. Serve the chia seed pudding with berries immediately as a nutritious and satisfying breakfast or dessert.

8. Enjoy the creamy texture of the chia seed pudding combined with the sweetness of the berries!

Chia seed pudding with berries is not only delicious but also packed with fiber, protein, and healthy fats. It's a great way to start your day or satisfy your sweet tooth while still enjoying a nutritious treat. Feel free to customize it with your favorite toppings or add-ins to suit your taste preferences!

81. Dark chocolate avocado mousse

Ingredients:
- 2 ripe avocados, peeled and pitted
- 1/4 cup cocoa powder
- 1/4 cup maple syrup or honey (adjust to taste)
- 1 teaspoon vanilla extract
- Pinch of salt
- Optional toppings: shaved dark chocolate, chopped nuts, fresh berries, whipped cream

Instructions:
1. In a food processor or blender, combine the ripe avocados, cocoa powder, maple syrup or honey, vanilla extract, and a pinch of salt.

2. Blend the ingredients until smooth and creamy, scraping down the sides of the bowl as needed to ensure everything is well combined.

3. Taste the mousse and adjust the sweetness if necessary by adding more maple syrup or honey.

4. Once the mousse reaches your desired consistency and sweetness, transfer it to serving bowls or glasses.

5. Cover the bowls or glasses with plastic wrap and refrigerate the mousse for at least 30 minutes to chill and firm up.

6. Optional: Before serving, garnish the dark chocolate avocado mousse with shaved dark chocolate, chopped nuts, fresh berries, or a dollop of whipped cream for added flavor and presentation.

7. Serve the dark chocolate avocado mousse chilled as a decadent and satisfying dessert.

8. Enjoy the velvety texture and rich chocolate flavor of this delicious and nutritious treat!

Dark chocolate avocado mousse is a great way to indulge your sweet tooth while still incorporating healthy fats and nutrients into your diet. It's vegan, gluten-free, and naturally sweetened, making it suitable for a variety of dietary preferences. Plus, it's so creamy and delicious that you won't even realize you're eating avocados!

82. Fresh fruit sorbet

Ingredients:
- 4 cups fresh fruit (such as berries, mango, pineapple, peaches, or a combination)
- 1/2 cup granulated sugar
- 1/4 cup water
- 1 tablespoon lemon juice (optional, for added freshness)

Instructions:
1. Wash and prepare the fresh fruit as needed. If using larger fruits like mango or pineapple, peel and chop them into chunks.

2. Place the fruit chunks in a blender or food processor and puree until smooth.

3. In a small saucepan, combine the granulated sugar and water. Heat over medium heat, stirring constantly, until the sugar is completely dissolved. This will create a simple syrup.

4. Once the sugar is dissolved, remove the saucepan from the heat and let the simple syrup cool to room temperature.

5. Once cooled, add the simple syrup and lemon juice (if using) to the fruit puree in the blender or food processor. Blend again until everything is well combined.

6. Taste the mixture and adjust the sweetness or acidity if needed by adding more sugar or lemon juice.

7. Pour the fruit mixture into a shallow baking dish or metal pan. Cover the dish with plastic wrap and place it in the freezer.

8. Every 30 minutes to an hour, remove the dish from the freezer and use a fork to scrape and stir the sorbet mixture. This will break up any ice crystals and create a smoother texture.

9. Continue to freeze and stir the sorbet mixture until it's firm and scoopable, usually about 3-4 hours total.

10. Once the sorbet is ready, scoop it into serving bowls or glasses and enjoy immediately as a refreshing treat. Store any leftover sorbet in an airtight container in the freezer for up to a few weeks.

Feel free to experiment with different combinations of fruits and add-ins to create your own unique sorbet flavors. You can also substitute honey or agave syrup for the granulated sugar for a different sweetness profile. Enjoy the fresh and vibrant flavors of homemade fruit sorbet!

83. Almond flour cookies

Ingredients:
- 2 cups almond flour
- 1/4 cup coconut oil or unsalted butter, melted
- 1/4 cup maple syrup or honey
- 1 teaspoon vanilla extract
- 1/4 teaspoon baking soda
- 1/4 teaspoon salt
- Optional add-ins: chocolate chips, chopped nuts, dried fruit

Instructions:
1. Preheat your oven to 350°F (175°C). Line a baking sheet with parchment paper or silicone baking mat.

2. In a large mixing bowl, combine the almond flour, melted coconut oil or butter, maple syrup or honey, vanilla extract, baking soda, and salt. Mix until everything is well combined and forms a dough.

3. If using any optional add-ins like chocolate chips or nuts, gently fold them into the cookie dough until evenly distributed.

4. Use a tablespoon or cookie scoop to portion out the dough and roll it into balls. Place the balls of dough onto the prepared baking sheet, leaving some space between each cookie.

5. Use a fork to gently flatten each cookie ball into a round disc shape.

6. Bake the cookies in the preheated oven for 10-12 minutes, or until the edges are golden brown.

7. Once baked, remove the cookies from the oven and let them cool on the baking sheet for a few minutes before transferring them to a wire rack to cool completely.

8. Enjoy the almond flour cookies as a delicious gluten-free treat!

These almond flour cookies are soft, chewy, and full of nutty flavor. They're perfect for satisfying your sweet tooth without the guilt, thanks to the wholesome ingredients like almond flour and natural sweeteners. Feel free to customize them with your favorite add-ins or spices to suit your taste preferences!

84. Banana and oat cookies

Ingredients:
- 2 ripe bananas, mashed
- 1 1/2 cups rolled oats (old-fashioned or quick oats)
- 1/4 cup nut butter (such as almond butter or peanut butter)
- 1/4 cup honey or maple syrup
- 1/2 teaspoon vanilla extract
- Optional add-ins: chocolate chips, chopped nuts, dried fruit, cinnamon

Instructions:
1. Preheat your oven to 350°F (175°C). Line a baking sheet with parchment paper or silicone baking mat.

2. In a large mixing bowl, combine the mashed bananas, rolled oats, nut butter, honey or maple syrup, and vanilla extract. Mix until everything is well combined and forms a sticky dough.

3. If using any optional add-ins like chocolate chips or nuts, gently fold them into the cookie dough until evenly distributed.

4. Use a tablespoon or cookie scoop to portion out the dough and drop it onto the prepared baking sheet, leaving some space between each cookie.

5. Use your fingers or the back of a spoon to flatten each cookie slightly, as they won't spread much during baking.

6. Bake the cookies in the preheated oven for 12-15 minutes, or until they are lightly golden brown around the edges.

7. Once baked, remove the cookies from the oven and let them cool on the baking sheet for a few minutes before transferring them to a wire rack to cool completely.

8. Enjoy the banana and oat cookies as a wholesome and satisfying snack!

These cookies are soft, chewy, and naturally sweetened by the ripe bananas and honey or maple syrup. They're packed with fiber, vitamins, and minerals from the oats and bananas, making them a nutritious choice for any time of day. Feel free to customize them with your favorite add-ins or spices to suit your taste preferences!

85. Mixed berry parfait with Greek yogurt

Ingredients:
- 1 cup mixed berries (such as strawberries, blueberries, raspberries)
- 1 cup Greek yogurt (plain or flavored)
- 1/4 cup granola
- 1 tablespoon honey or maple syrup (optional, for sweetness)
- Fresh mint leaves for garnish (optional)

Instructions:
1. Wash the mixed berries and pat them dry. If using strawberries, hull and slice them.

2. In a small bowl or glass, layer the ingredients starting with a spoonful of Greek yogurt at the bottom.

3. Add a layer of mixed berries on top of the yogurt.

4. Sprinkle a layer of granola over the mixed berries.

5. Repeat the layers until you reach the top of the bowl or glass, finishing with a final layer of Greek yogurt.

6. If desired, drizzle honey or maple syrup over the top for added sweetness.

7. Garnish the parfait with fresh mint leaves for a pop of color and freshness.

8. Serve the mixed berry parfait immediately as a delicious and nutritious breakfast or dessert.

Mixed berry parfait with Greek yogurt is not only delicious but also packed with protein, fiber, and antioxidants. It's a great way to start your day or satisfy your sweet tooth while still enjoying a wholesome treat. Feel free to customize it with your favorite berries, yogurt flavors, or additional toppings like chopped nuts or coconut flakes!

86. Coconut milk ice cream

Ingredients:
- 1 cup mixed berries (such as strawberries, blueberries, raspberries)
- 1 cup Greek yogurt (plain or flavored)
- 1/4 cup granola
- 1 tablespoon honey or maple syrup (optional, for sweetness)
- Fresh mint leaves for garnish (optional)

Instructions:
1. Wash the mixed berries and pat them dry. If using strawberries, hull and slice them.

2. In a small bowl or glass, layer the ingredients starting with a spoonful of Greek yogurt at the bottom.

3. Add a layer of mixed berries on top of the yogurt.

4. Sprinkle a layer of granola over the mixed berries.

5. Repeat the layers until you reach the top of the bowl or glass, finishing with a final layer of Greek yogurt.

6. If desired, drizzle honey or maple syrup over the top for added sweetness.

7. Garnish the parfait with fresh mint leaves for a pop of color and freshness.

8. Serve the mixed berry parfait immediately as a delicious and nutritious breakfast or dessert.

Mixed berry parfait with Greek yogurt is not only delicious but also packed with protein, fiber, and antioxidants. It's a great way to start your day or satisfy your sweet tooth while still enjoying a wholesome treat. Feel free to customize it with your favorite berries, yogurt flavors, or additional toppings like chopped nuts or coconut flakes!

87. Stewed fruit with a dollop of yogurt

Ingredients:
- 2 cups mixed fruit (such as apples, pears, peaches, plums, or berries), peeled and chopped if necessary
- 2 tablespoons honey or maple syrup
- 1 teaspoon ground cinnamon
- 1/2 teaspoon vanilla extract
- 1 cup Greek yogurt (plain or flavored)

Instructions:

1. In a medium saucepan, combine the mixed fruit, honey or maple syrup, ground cinnamon, and vanilla extract.

2. Cook the fruit mixture over medium heat, stirring occasionally, until the fruit is soft and begins to release its juices. This will take about 5-10 minutes, depending on the type of fruit you're using.

3. Once the fruit is stewed to your liking, remove the saucepan from the heat and let it cool slightly.

4. Spoon the stewed fruit into serving bowls or glasses.

5. Top each serving of stewed fruit with a dollop of Greek yogurt.

6. Serve the stewed fruit with a dollop of yogurt immediately as a delicious and wholesome dessert or breakfast.

7. Enjoy the warm and comforting flavors of the stewed fruit paired with the creamy richness of the yogurt!

Stewed fruit with a dollop of yogurt is not only delicious but also packed with vitamins, fiber, and protein. It's a great way to enjoy seasonal fruits and add variety to your breakfast or dessert routine. Feel free to customize it with your favorite fruits, spices, or additional toppings like chopped nuts or granola for added texture and flavor.

88. Avocado chocolate pudding

Ingredients:
- 2 ripe avocados, peeled and pitted
- 1/2 cup cocoa powder
- 1/2 cup maple syrup or honey
- 1/4 cup almond milk or any milk of your choice
- 1 teaspoon vanilla extract
- Pinch of salt
- Optional toppings: shaved dark chocolate, chopped nuts, fresh berries, whipped cream

Instructions:
1. In a food processor or blender, combine the ripe avocados, cocoa powder, maple syrup or honey, almond milk, vanilla extract, and a pinch of salt.

2. Blend the ingredients until smooth and creamy, scraping down the sides of the bowl as needed to ensure everything is well combined.

3. Taste the pudding and adjust the sweetness or thickness if necessary by adding more maple syrup, cocoa powder, or almond milk.

4. Once the pudding reaches your desired consistency and sweetness, transfer it to serving bowls or glasses.

5. Cover the bowls or glasses with plastic wrap and refrigerate the pudding for at least 30 minutes to chill and firm up.

6. Optional: Before serving, garnish the avocado chocolate pudding with shaved dark chocolate, chopped nuts, fresh berries, or a dollop of whipped cream for added flavor and presentation.

7. Serve the avocado chocolate pudding chilled as a decadent and satisfying dessert.

8. Enjoy the rich and velvety texture of this delicious and nutritious treat!

Avocado chocolate pudding is a great way to satisfy your sweet tooth while still incorporating healthy fats and nutrients into your diet. It's vegan, gluten-free, and naturally sweetened, making it suitable for a variety of dietary preferences. Plus, it's so creamy and delicious that you won't even realize you're eating avocados! Feel free to customize it with your favorite toppings or add-ins to suit your taste preferences!

89. Kefir smoothie with berries

Ingredients:
- 1 cup kefir (plain or flavored)
- 1 cup mixed berries (such as strawberries, blueberries, raspberries)
- 1 ripe banana, fresh or frozen
- 1 tablespoon honey or maple syrup (optional, for added sweetness)
- Handful of ice cubes (optional, for a colder smoothie)
- Optional add-ins: spinach or kale for extra greens, chia seeds or flaxseeds for added fiber and omega-3s, protein powder for added protein

Instructions:
1. In a blender, combine the kefir, mixed berries, ripe banana, and honey or maple syrup (if using).

2. If you prefer a colder smoothie, add a handful of ice cubes to the blender as well.

3. Blend the ingredients until smooth and creamy, adjusting the consistency by adding more kefir or ice cubes as needed.

4. Taste the smoothie and adjust the sweetness if necessary by adding more honey or maple syrup.

5. Once the smoothie reaches your desired consistency and sweetness, pour it into serving glasses.

6. Optional: Garnish the smoothie with additional berries or a sprig of fresh mint for added freshness and presentation.

7. Serve the kefir smoothie with berries immediately as a delicious and nutritious breakfast or snack.

8. Enjoy the creamy texture and vibrant flavors of this refreshing smoothie!

Kefir smoothie with berries is not only tasty but also packed with probiotics, vitamins, and antioxidants. It's a great way to support gut health and boost your immune system while enjoying a delicious and satisfying treat. Feel free to customize it with your favorite fruits, greens, or add-ins to suit your taste preferences and nutritional needs!

90. Green tea

Ingredients:
- 1 teaspoon green tea leaves (or 1 tea bag)
- 1 cup hot water (about 175°F or 80°C)

Instructions:
1. Bring water to a boil and then let it cool for a few minutes until it reaches about 175°F (80°C). This temperature is ideal for green tea to avoid bitterness.

2. Place the green tea leaves in a teapot or a cup. If using a tea bag, simply place the tea bag in the cup.

3. Pour the hot water over the green tea leaves or tea bag.

4. Let the tea steep for about 2-3 minutes. Steeping too long can result in a bitter taste, so it's best to start with a shorter steeping time and adjust to your preference.

5. Once the tea has steeped, remove the tea leaves or tea bag from the cup.

6. If desired, you can add honey, lemon, or a slice of fresh ginger to enhance the flavor of the green tea.

7. Serve the green tea hot and enjoy its soothing taste and health benefits.

Green tea is rich in antioxidants and has been associated with various health benefits, including improved brain function, fat loss, and reduced risk of certain cancers. It's also low in calories and can be enjoyed throughout the day as a refreshing beverage. Feel free to experiment with different varieties of green tea, such as sencha, matcha, or genmaicha, to find your favorite flavor!

91. Kombucha

Ingredients:
- SCOBY
- Starter tea
- Water
- Sugar
- Tea (black, green, or white)

Brewing Process:
1. Brew tea and dissolve sugar in it.

2. Cool the sweetened tea and transfer to a clean jar.

3. Add SCOBY and starter tea to the jar.

4. Cover and ferment for 7-14 days.

Flavoring and Bottling:

1. Remove SCOBY and some liquid for next batch.

2. Optionally, flavor kombucha with fruit juice or spices.

3. Let it ferment for 1-7 days.

4. Strain out solids and bottle in clean containers.

5. Let bottles carbonate for 1-3 days at room temperature.

6. Refrigerate before serving.

Enjoy your homemade kombucha for its probiotic benefits and refreshing taste!

92. Lemon water

Ingredients:
- 1-inch piece of fresh ginger, sliced
- 2 bay leaves
- 1 tablespoon apple cider vinegar
(helps extract minerals from the bones)
- Salt and pepper to taste
- Water
- 2-3 pounds beef or chicken bones
(such as marrow bones, knuckles, or
neck bones)
- 1 onion, peeled and halved
- 2 carrots, chopped
- 2 celery stalks, chopped
- 3-4 cloves garlic, smashed

Instructions:
1. Preheat your oven to 400°F (200°C). Place the bones on a baking sheet and roast in the oven for about 30 minutes, or until they are browned and fragrant. This step helps deepen the flavor of the broth.

2. Transfer the roasted bones to a large stockpot or slow cooker. Add the onion, carrots, celery, garlic, ginger, bay leaves, and apple cider vinegar to the pot.

3. Fill the pot with enough water to cover the bones and vegetables completely. Add salt and pepper to taste.

4. If using a stockpot, bring the mixture to a boil over high heat. Once boiling, reduce the heat to low and let the broth simmer gently for at least 6-8 hours, or up to 24 hours for maximum flavor and nutrient extraction. Skim off any foam or impurities that rise to the surface during simmering.

   If using a slow cooker, set it to low heat and let the broth cook for 8-24 hours.

5. Once the broth has finished cooking, remove the bones and vegetables with a slotted spoon and discard them. Strain the broth through a fine mesh sieve or cheesecloth to remove any remaining solids.

6. Let the broth cool slightly before transferring it to storage containers. Store the broth in the refrigerator for up to 5 days, or freeze it for longer storage. Serve the bone broth with ginger and garlic hot as a comforting and nourishing soup.

Bone broth with ginger and garlic is rich in nutrients and minerals, making it a great addition to your diet for supporting gut health and immune function. Enjoy it on its own or use it as a base for soups, stews, and sauces. Adjust the seasonings and add-ins to suit your taste preferences!

93. Fresh vegetable juice

Ingredients:
- 2 large carrots
- 2 stalks celery
- 1 cucumber
- 1 small beet
- 1 handful spinach or kale
- 1/2 lemon, peeled
- Optional: ginger root (about 1-inch piece), parsley, cilantro

Instructions:
1. Wash all the vegetables thoroughly.

2. Trim the ends off the carrots, celery, and cucumber. Peel the beet and chop it into smaller pieces if necessary.

3. Cut the vegetables into sizes that will fit into your juicer chute.

4. Juice the vegetables and lemon in a juicer according to the manufacturer's instructions. Start with the softer vegetables like spinach or cucumber, followed by harder vegetables like carrots and beets.

5. If using ginger, pass it through the juicer with the other vegetables.

6. Once all the vegetables are juiced, give the juice a good stir to combine.

7. Taste the juice and adjust the flavor by adding more lemon or ginger if desired.

8. Serve the fresh vegetable juice immediately over ice for a refreshing drink.

Fresh vegetable juice is a great way to hydrate your body and pack in essential nutrients from a variety of vegetables. It's naturally low in calories and high in vitamins, minerals, and antioxidants. Feel free to customize the recipe with your favorite vegetables and herbs to suit your taste preferences and nutritional needs!

94. Ginger tea

Ingredients:
- 1-inch piece of fresh ginger root
- 2 cups water
- Optional: honey, lemon slices, or mint leaves for flavor

Instructions:

1. Peel the ginger root and slice it thinly or grate it using a fine grater.

2. In a small saucepan, bring the water to a boil.

3. Add the sliced or grated ginger to the boiling water.

4. Reduce the heat to low and let the ginger simmer in the water for about 5-10 minutes, depending on how strong you like your ginger tea.

5. Once the tea has reached your desired strength, remove the saucepan from the heat.

6. If desired, strain the ginger pieces from the tea using a fine mesh sieve or cheesecloth.

7. Pour the ginger tea into serving cups.

8. Optionally, add honey, lemon slices, or mint leaves to flavor the tea.

9. Serve the ginger tea hot for immediate enjoyment, or let it cool and refrigerate for a refreshing iced tea.

Ginger tea is known for its warming and soothing properties, making it a great choice for cold winter days or to calm an upset stomach. It's naturally caffeine-free and low in calories, making it a healthy beverage option. Experiment with different flavor additions like cinnamon or cloves to create your own unique ginger tea blend!

95. Herbal tea blends

Ingredients:
- Base herbs: Choose one or more base herbs for the foundation of your blend. Some popular options include:
  - Peppermint
  - Chamomile
  - Rooibos
  - Lemongrass
  - Lemon balm
  - Hibiscus
  - Green tea (for a slight caffeine boost)
- Optional medicinal herbs: If you're looking to create a blend with specific health benefits, consider adding medicinal herbs such as:
  - Echinacea
  - Elderflower
  - Nettle leaf
  - Dandelion root
  - Licorice root
  - Astragalus
  - Ashwagandha

- Flavoring herbs: Add flavor and depth to your blend with additional herbs and spices. Some ideas include:
  - Lavender, Ginger, Cinnamon, Cardamom, Fennel seeds, Orange peel, Rose petals

Instructions:

1. Start by selecting your base herbs and any additional flavoring or medicinal herbs you'd like to include in your blend.

2. Experiment with different combinations and proportions of herbs until you find a flavor profile that you enjoy. You can mix and match herbs to create unique flavor combinations.

3. Once you've settled on your desired blend, combine the herbs in a mixing bowl or jar. Use about 1-2 teaspoons of herbs per cup of tea.

4. Store your herbal tea blend in an airtight container away from light and heat to preserve its freshness.

5. To brew the tea, simply place 1-2 teaspoons of the herbal blend in a tea infuser or teapot and pour hot water over it. Let it steep for 5-10 minutes, then strain and enjoy.

6. Feel free to adjust the strength of the tea by adding more or less of the herbal blend, and experiment with steeping times to achieve your preferred flavor intensity.

7. Get creative and personalize your herbal tea blends to suit your taste preferences and health goals. Whether you're looking for a relaxing bedtime tea, a refreshing afternoon pick-me-up, or a soothing remedy for a sore throat, there's a blend for every occasion!

Creating your own herbal tea blends allows you to tailor the flavor and benefits to your liking, and it's a fun and rewarding way to explore the world of herbalism. So gather your favorite herbs and spices, and start blending!

96. Coconut water

Instructions:
1. Choose a fresh, young coconut or purchase packaged coconut water from the grocery store. Look for brands that offer 100% pure coconut water without added sugars or preservatives.

2. If using a fresh coconut, carefully use a sharp knife to cut through the husk and crack it open. Pour the coconut water into a clean glass or container.

3. If using packaged coconut water, simply open the container or bottle and pour the coconut water into a glass.

4. Serve the coconut water chilled over ice for a refreshing drink.

5. Optionally, you can add a squeeze of lime or lemon juice for extra flavor, or garnish with a slice of citrus.

6. Enjoy the coconut water on its own as a hydrating beverage, or use it as a base for smoothies, cocktails, or mocktails.

Coconut water is naturally rich in potassium, magnesium, and other electrolytes, making it an excellent choice for replenishing fluids and rehydrating after exercise or on hot days. It's also low in sugar and calories, making it a healthier alternative to sugary drinks. So sit back, relax, and enjoy the tropical taste and benefits of coconut water!

97. Water infused with cucumber and mint

Ingredients:
- 1 cucumber, washed and sliced
- 1 handful fresh mint leaves, washed
- Water

Instructions:

1. Place the cucumber slices and mint leaves in a large pitcher or glass jar.

2. Fill the pitcher or jar with water, covering the cucumber slices and mint leaves completely.

3. Stir the water gently to release the flavors of the cucumber and mint.

4. Refrigerate the infused water for at least 1-2 hours, or overnight for stronger flavor.

5. Once infused, strain out the cucumber slices and mint leaves if desired, or leave them in the water for added visual appeal.

6. Serve the cucumber and mint infused water chilled over ice for a refreshing and hydrating drink.

7. Optionally, you can garnish individual glasses with additional cucumber slices and mint leaves for a decorative touch.

Cucumber and mint infused water is a healthy and flavorful alternative to sugary beverages, and it's perfect for staying hydrated throughout the day. Enjoy it on its own or alongside meals for a refreshing palate cleanser. Feel free to customize the recipe with other fruits or herbs like lemon, lime, or basil for endless flavor combinations!

98. Bone broth

Ingredients:
- 1 onion, peeled and halved
- 3-4 cloves garlic, smashed
- 2 bay leaves
- 1 tablespoon apple cider vinegar
  (helps extract minerals from the bones)
- Salt and pepper to taste
- Water
- 2-3 pounds beef, chicken, or pork bones (such as marrow bones, knuckles, or neck bones)
- 2 carrots, chopped
- 2 celery stalks, chopped

Instructions:

1. Preheat your oven to 400°F (200°C). Place the bones on a baking sheet and roast in the oven for about 30 minutes, or until they are browned and fragrant. This step helps deepen the flavor of the broth.

2. Transfer the roasted bones to a large stockpot or slow cooker. Add the chopped carrots, celery, onion, garlic, bay leaves, and apple cider vinegar to the pot.

3. Fill the pot with enough water to cover the bones and vegetables completely.

4. If using a stockpot, bring the mixture to a boil over high heat. Once boiling, reduce the heat to low and let the broth simmer gently for at least 6-8 hours, or up to 24 hours for maximum flavor and nutrient extraction. Skim off any foam or impurities that rise to the surface during simmering.

   If using a slow cooker, set it to low heat and let the broth cook for 8-24 hours.

5. Once the broth has finished cooking, remove the bones and vegetables with a slotted spoon and discard them. Strain the broth through a fine mesh sieve or cheesecloth to remove any remaining solids.

6. Let the broth cool slightly before transferring it to storage containers. Store the broth in the refrigerator for up to 5 days, or freeze it for longer storage.

7. Use the bone broth as a base for soups, stews, sauces, or enjoy it on its own as a nourishing and comforting drink.

Bone broth is rich in vitamins, minerals, and collagen, making it a nutritious addition to your diet. It's also a great way to use up leftover bones and vegetable scraps, reducing food waste. Feel free to customize the recipe with your favorite herbs and spices to suit your taste preferences!

99. Chamomile tea

Ingredients:
- 1-2 teaspoons dried chamomile flowers or 1 chamomile tea bag
- 1 cup water

Instructions:

1. Boil water in a kettle or saucepan.

2. Place the chamomile flowers or tea bag in a cup or teapot.

3. Pour the boiling water over the chamomile flowers or tea bag.

4. Let the tea steep for about 5 minutes to allow the flavors to infuse.

5. Remove the chamomile flowers or tea bag from the cup or teapot.

6. Optionally, you can add honey, lemon, or a slice of orange for extra flavor.

7. Stir the tea gently and taste. Adjust the sweetness or acidity as desired.

8. Serve the chamomile tea hot and enjoy its calming and relaxing effects.

Chamomile tea is caffeine-free and is often consumed before bedtime to promote relaxation and improve sleep quality. It's also known for its mild, floral flavor, making it a delightful beverage to enjoy at any time of day. Feel free to experiment with steeping times and flavor additions to customize your chamomile tea to your liking!

100. Turmeric latte

Ingredients:
- 1 cup milk of your choice (dairy milk, almond milk, coconut milk, etc.)
- 1 teaspoon ground turmeric
- 1/2 teaspoon ground cinnamon
- 1/4 teaspoon ground ginger
- Pinch of black pepper (helps with the absorption of turmeric)
- Pinch of ground nutmeg (optional)
- Sweetener of your choice, such as honey, maple syrup, or stevia (optional)

Instructions:
1. In a small saucepan, heat the milk over medium-low heat until it begins to steam. Be careful not to let it boil.

2. Add the ground turmeric, cinnamon, ginger, black pepper, and nutmeg to the milk.

3. Whisk the ingredients together until well combined.

4. Continue to heat the mixture for another 3-5 minutes, stirring occasionally, until it is hot but not boiling.

5. Remove the saucepan from the heat and taste the turmeric latte. If desired, add sweetener to taste and stir until dissolved.

6. Pour the turmeric latte into a mug and serve immediately.

7. Optionally, you can garnish the turmeric latte with a sprinkle of ground cinnamon or a cinnamon stick for extra flavor and visual appeal.

Turmeric latte is not only delicious but also packed with antioxidants and anti-inflammatory properties thanks to the turmeric. It's a comforting and nourishing beverage that's perfect for cozy evenings or as a caffeine-free alternative to coffee. Feel free to adjust the spices and sweetness to suit your taste preferences!

101. Aloe vera juice

Ingredients:
- Fresh aloe vera leaf
- Water
- Optional: lemon juice, honey, or other sweeteners for flavor

Instructions:
1. Wash the aloe vera leaf thoroughly under running water to remove any dirt or debris.

2. Using a sharp knife, carefully slice off the serrated edges of the aloe vera leaf.

3. Cut the aloe vera leaf into smaller sections, then slice each section lengthwise to expose the inner gel.

4. Scoop out the gel from the aloe vera leaf using a spoon and transfer it to a blender or food processor.

5. Add water to the blender at a ratio of about 1 cup of water for every 2 tablespoons of aloe vera gel.

6. Blend the mixture until smooth and well combined.

7. Optionally, you can strain the aloe vera juice through a fine mesh sieve or cheesecloth to remove any remaining pulp.

8. Add lemon juice, honey, or other sweeteners to taste, if desired, and stir until dissolved.

9. Transfer the aloe vera juice to a clean glass jar or bottle for storage.

10. Refrigerate the aloe vera juice for up to 1 week.

Aloe vera juice is known for its potential digestive and skin health benefits, thanks to its anti-inflammatory and soothing properties. It's best consumed in moderation, as excessive consumption may have laxative effects for some individuals. Enjoy a small glass of aloe vera juice on its own or mixed with other juices for added flavor and nutrients!

102. Kimchi

Ingredients:
- 1 medium Napa cabbage
- 1 daikon radish (or Korean radish)
- 1/4 cup sea salt
- 2 tablespoons Korean red pepper flakes (gochugaru)
- Water
- 3 cloves garlic, minced
- 1 tablespoon grated ginger
- 2 tablespoons fish sauce (or soy sauce for a vegetarian version)
- 2 green onions, chopped
- 1 tablespoon sugar (optional)
- 1 tablespoon rice flour (optional, to help with fermentation)

Instructions:

1. Cut the Napa cabbage lengthwise into quarters, then remove the core. Chop the cabbage into bite-sized pieces.

2. Peel the daikon radish and cut it into thin matchsticks or slices.

3. In a large bowl, dissolve the sea salt in water to create a brine. Add the chopped cabbage and radish to the brine, making sure they are fully submerged. Let them soak for 1-2 hours.

4. Rinse the cabbage and radish under cold water to remove excess salt. Drain well and set aside.

5. In a separate bowl, combine the Korean red pepper flakes, minced garlic, grated ginger, fish sauce (or soy sauce), chopped green onions, sugar (if using), and rice flour (if using).

6. Add the drained cabbage and radish to the spice mixture. Use your hands to massage the spice mixture into the vegetables, ensuring they are well coated.

7. Pack the kimchi tightly into clean glass jars or fermentation crocks, pressing down to remove any air bubbles.

8. Cover the jars or crocks loosely with lids or clean towels to allow for fermentation. Let the kimchi ferment at room temperature for 1-5 days, depending on your preference for taste and texture. The longer it ferments, the more sour and tangy it will become.

9. Once fermented to your liking, seal the jars or crocks tightly and store the kimchi in the refrigerator. It will continue to ferment slowly in the fridge, developing deeper flavors over time. Enjoy homemade kimchi as a side dish, condiment, or ingredient in various Korean dishes!

Kimchi is not only delicious but also packed with probiotics and nutrients, making it a healthy addition to your diet. Feel free to customize the recipe with additional vegetables or spices to suit your taste preferences!

103. Sauerkraut

Ingredients:
- 1 medium head of cabbage (green or red)
- 1 1/2 tablespoons sea salt
- Optional: caraway seeds, juniper berries, or other spices for flavor

Instructions:

1. Remove the outer leaves of the cabbage and set them aside. Cut the cabbage into quarters and remove the core.

2. Thinly slice the cabbage into shreds using a knife or mandoline.

3. Place the shredded cabbage in a large bowl and sprinkle the sea salt over the top.

4. Use your hands to massage the salt into the cabbage for a few minutes. This helps to release the juices from the cabbage and start the fermentation process.

5. Let the cabbage sit for about 10-15 minutes to allow more liquid to be released.

6. Pack the cabbage tightly into clean glass jars or fermentation crocks, pressing down to submerge the cabbage under its own juices. If there isn't enough liquid to cover the cabbage, you can top it off with a bit of water mixed with salt (about 1 teaspoon of salt per cup of water).

7. If desired, sprinkle caraway seeds, juniper berries, or other spices over the top of the cabbage for added flavor.

8. Place the reserved cabbage leaves on top of the shredded cabbage to help keep it submerged.

9. Cover the jars or crocks loosely with lids or clean towels to allow for fermentation. Let the sauerkraut ferment at room temperature for 3-10 days, depending on your preference for taste and texture. The longer it ferments, the tangier it will become.

10. Once fermented to your liking, seal the jars or crocks tightly and store the sauerkraut in the refrigerator. It will continue to ferment slowly in the fridge, developing deeper flavors over time. Enjoy homemade sauerkraut as a side dish, condiment, or ingredient in various dishes!

Sauerkraut is not only tasty but also packed with probiotics and nutrients, making it a healthy addition to your diet. Feel free to experiment with different cabbage varieties and spices to customize the flavor to your liking!

104. Pickled cucumbers

Ingredients:
- 3-4 cucumbers (Kirby or pickling cucumbers work best)
- 2 cups water
- 1 cup white vinegar
- 2 tablespoons salt
- 2 cloves garlic, peeled and smashed
- 1 teaspoon whole black peppercorns
- 1 teaspoon mustard seeds
- 1 teaspoon dill seeds (optional)
- 1 teaspoon red pepper flakes (optional)
- 1 bay leaf (optional)
- Fresh dill sprigs (optional)

Instructions:
1. Wash the cucumbers thoroughly and trim off the ends. Slice the cucumbers into rounds or spears, depending on your preference.

2. In a saucepan, combine the water, vinegar, salt, garlic, peppercorns, mustard seeds, dill seeds, red pepper flakes, and bay leaf. Bring the mixture to a boil, then reduce the heat and simmer for about 5 minutes to infuse the flavors.

3. Pack the cucumber slices or spears into clean glass jars, leaving about 1/2 inch of space at the top.

4. Pour the hot brine over the cucumbers in the jars, covering them completely. If using, add a few sprigs of fresh dill to each jar for extra flavor.

5. Use a clean spoon to press down on the cucumbers to remove any air bubbles and ensure they are fully submerged in the brine.

6. Seal the jars tightly with lids and let them cool to room temperature.

7. Once cooled, transfer the jars to the refrigerator and let the pickles chill for at least 24 hours before serving. The longer they sit, the more flavorful they will become.

8. Enjoy homemade pickled cucumbers as a tangy and crunchy snack, or use them as a topping for sandwiches, salads, burgers, and more!

Pickled cucumbers are a versatile and delicious addition to your pantry, and they're easy to customize with different herbs and spices. Feel free to experiment with the flavorings to create your own unique pickle recipe!

105. Miso soup

Ingredients:
- 4 cups dashi broth (or vegetable broth for a vegetarian version)
- 3 tablespoons miso paste (white or red)
- 1 block firm tofu, cut into small cubes
- 2 green onions, thinly sliced
- 1 sheet nori (dried seaweed), cut into thin strips
- Optional: sliced mushrooms, spinach, cooked shrimp, or other additions of your choice

Instructions:
1. In a saucepan, bring the dashi broth to a gentle simmer over medium heat.

2. In a small bowl, dilute the miso paste with a few tablespoons of hot broth to make it easier to mix.

3. Add the diluted miso paste to the simmering broth and stir well to combine. Let the soup simmer for a few minutes to allow the flavors to meld.

4. Add the cubed tofu to the soup and simmer for another 2-3 minutes, or until heated through.

5. Add any additional ingredients you'd like, such as sliced mushrooms, spinach, or cooked shrimp, and simmer until they are cooked to your liking.

6. Remove the soup from the heat and stir in the sliced green onions and nori strips.

7. Taste the soup and adjust the seasoning if necessary, adding more miso paste for a stronger flavor or more broth to dilute.

8. Serve the miso soup hot in individual bowls and enjoy as a comforting and nourishing meal.

Miso soup is a versatile dish that can be customized with various ingredients to suit your taste preferences and dietary needs. Feel free to experiment with different vegetables, proteins, and types of miso paste to create your own unique version of this classic Japanese soup!

106. Tempeh

Ingredients:
- 1 block tempeh
- Marinade or seasoning of your choice (such as soy sauce, tamari, garlic, ginger, maple syrup, or chili flakes)

Instructions:

1. Cut the tempeh into slices or cubes, depending on how you plan to use it.

2. If desired, you can steam the tempeh for about 10 minutes to reduce its bitterness and help it absorb flavors better. Alternatively, you can skip this step if you prefer a firmer texture.

3. Prepare a marinade or seasoning of your choice. Popular options include soy sauce or tamari, minced garlic, grated ginger, maple syrup or honey for sweetness, and chili flakes for heat. Feel free to customize the marinade to suit your taste preferences.

4. Place the tempeh slices or cubes in a shallow dish or zip-top bag, and pour the marinade over them. Make sure the tempeh is evenly coated with the marinade.

5. Let the tempeh marinate for at least 30 minutes, or ideally for a few hours or overnight in the refrigerator. This allows the flavors to penetrate the tempeh and enhance its taste.

6. After marinating, you can cook the tempeh using your preferred method. It can be pan-fried, baked, grilled, or sautéed until golden brown and crispy on the outside and heated through.

7. Serve the cooked tempeh as a protein-rich main dish or as a topping for salads, sandwiches, stir-fries, or grain bowls.

Tempeh is a nutritious plant-based source of protein, fiber, and vitamins. It absorbs flavors well, making it a versatile ingredient in various savory dishes. Experiment with different marinades, seasonings, and cooking methods to discover your favorite way to enjoy tempeh!

107. Natto

Ingredients:
- Natto (available at Japanese or Asian grocery stores)
- Prepared mustard (included with some packages of natto)
- Soy sauce or tamari
- Optional toppings: chopped green onions, grated daikon radish, shredded nori (seaweed), raw egg

Instructions:

1. Remove the natto from its packaging and transfer it to a bowl.

2. If the package includes prepared mustard, add it to the bowl. This helps to enhance the flavor of the natto.

3. Add soy sauce or tamari to the bowl, according to your taste preferences. Start with a small amount and adjust as needed.

4. Use chopsticks or a fork to mix the natto, mustard, and soy sauce together until well combined. The mixture will become sticky and stringy due to the fermentation process.

5. Optional: Add any desired toppings to the natto mixture, such as chopped green onions, grated daikon radish, shredded nori, or a raw egg.

6. Serve the natto as is, or enjoy it as a topping for rice or other grains.

Natto is known for its strong flavor and aroma, which may not be to everyone's taste. However, it's a nutritious food that's rich in protein, fiber, and probiotics. If you're new to natto, you may want to start with a small amount and gradually increase your intake as you become accustomed to its unique taste and texture.

108. Kombucha

Ingredients:
- 1 SCOBY (Symbiotic Culture Of Bacteria and Yeast)
- 1 cup starter tea (previously brewed kombucha)
- Tea (4-6 tea bags or 2-3 tablespoons loose leaf tea)
- 1 cup granulated sugar
- 3.5 liters (about 14 cups) filtered water
- Optional flavorings: fruit juice, ginger, herbs, spices, etc.

Instructions:
1. Brew tea, dissolve sugar, and cool to room temperature.

2. Combine tea, SCOBY, and starter tea in a clean jar.

3. Cover with cloth, secure, and ferment for 7-14 days.

4. Taste for desired acidity and carbonation.

5. Remove SCOBY, strain, and refrigerate.

6. Optionally flavor and ferment for 1-3 more days.

7. Chill and enjoy your homemade kombucha!

109. Fermented pickles

Ingredients:
- Pickling cucumbers
- Water
- Salt
- Garlic cloves
- Fresh dill
- Optional: spices like mustard seeds, peppercorns, or red pepper flakes

Instructions:
1. Wash cucumbers and pack them into clean jars along with garlic cloves and fresh dill.

2. Make a brine by dissolving salt in water (about 1-2 tablespoons of salt per quart of water).

3. Pour brine over cucumbers, ensuring they're fully submerged.

4. Add optional spices for flavor.

5. Cover jars loosely and let them ferment at room temperature for 3-7 days.

6. Taste pickles to check for desired sourness, then refrigerate to slow fermentation.

7. Enjoy your tangy homemade fermented pickles!

110. Fermented beets

Ingredients:
- Beets, peeled and sliced or grated
- Water
- Salt
- Optional: garlic cloves, ginger slices, or spices like coriander seeds or caraway seeds

Instructions:
1. Pack sliced or grated beets into clean jars, along with any optional flavorings like garlic, ginger, or spices.

2. Make a brine by dissolving salt in water (about 1-2 tablespoons of salt per quart of water).
3. Pour the brine over the beets, ensuring they're fully submerged.

4. Cover the jars loosely to allow gases to escape during fermentation.

5. Let the beets ferment at room temperature for 3-7 days, tasting occasionally for desired sourness.

6. Once fermented to your liking, refrigerate the beets to slow fermentation.

7. Enjoy your tangy homemade fermented beets as a tasty snack or addition to salads and sandwiches!

*As you reach the end of **"Manly Meals for Gut Health,"** I hope you've discovered more than just a collection of recipes. This book is a testament to the idea that taking care of your gut doesn't mean sacrificing the flavors and satisfaction you crave as a man. It's about embracing a lifestyle that nourishes your body from within while still indulging in the bold, hearty meals you love.*

Throughout these pages, we've explored the intricate connection between what we eat and how we feel, delving into the importance of gut health and providing practical tips for incorporating gut-friendly ingredients into your everyday meals. But more than that, we've celebrated the joy of cooking and the pleasure of sharing delicious, wholesome food with loved ones.

As you continue your journey towards optimal health, remember that every meal is an opportunity to nourish your body and support your well-being. Whether you're starting your day with a protein-packed breakfast, enjoying a satisfying lunch on the go, or savoring a hearty dinner with friends and family, let "Manly Meals for Gut Health" be your guide to making mindful, delicious choices that leave you feeling energized and fulfilled.

So, here's to good food, good health, and the good times that come from sharing both with those we care about. May your kitchen always be filled with laughter, flavor, and the comforting aroma of a meal made with love. Thank you for joining me on this culinary journey – may your gut be healthy and your meals always manly.